Colby, Kerr, and Robinson's
Color Atlas of
Oral Pathology

Fifth Edition   *478 Figures in Color*

Hamilton B. G. Robinson
D.D.S., M.S., D.Sc. (Hon.)
Dean Emeritus and Professor Emeritus
University of Missouri–Kansas City School of Dentistry
Kansas City, Missouri

Arthur S. Miller
D.M.D., M.S.D.
Professor of Pathology
Temple University School of Medicine
Philadelphia, Pennsylvania

J.B. Lippincott Company
Philadelphia • Grand Rapids • New York • St. Louis • San Francisco
London • Sydney • Tokyo

Colby, Kerr, and Robinson's
Color Atlas of Oral Pathology

Acquisitions Editor: Darlene Barela Cooke
Sponsoring Editor: Delois Patterson
Project Editor: Lorraine D. Smith
Manuscript Editor: Patrick O'Kane
Art Director: Susan Hess Blaker
Design Coordinator: Ellen C. Dawson
Cover Designer: Ellen C. Dawson
Production Manager: Carol Florence
Production Coordinator: Kevin P. Johnson
Compositor: Circle Graphics
Printer/Binder: R.R. Donnelley & Sons Company

6   5   4   3   2   1

Library of Congress Cataloging-in-Publication Data
Library of Congress Cataloging-in-Publication Data is available. LC card number
89–14038

ISBN 0-397-51043-8

The authors and publisher have exerted every effort to ensure that drug selection and
dosage set forth in this text are in accord with current recommendations and practice
at the time of publication. However, in view of ongoing research, changes in
government regulations, and the constant flow of information relating to drug therapy
and drug reactions, the reader is urged to check the package insert for each drug for
any change in indications and dosage and for added warnings and precautions. This is
particularly important when the recommended agent is a new or infrequently
employed drug.

Preface

The first edition of *Colby, Kerr, and Robinson's Color Atlas of Oral Pathology,* prepared under the auspices of the dental division of the United States Navy, was designed to offer a concise, pictorial reference guide from which knowledge could be readily gained. The text was clear, succinct, and authoritative. Subsequent editions, including this fifth edition, have perpetuated this original concept, while always updating all technical elements.

The authors, with the cooperation of the publisher, have thoroughly revised the Atlas. The chapter on diseases of the oral mucosa and jaws has been divided into two parts, one on inflammatory, infectious, and reactive lesions and the other on conditions resulting from altered immune states. The latter was prompted by newer knowledge of immune states and by the advent of AIDS and AIDS-related diseases affecting the oral regions. In addition, chapters on non-neoplastic conditions of bone and on genetic, metabolic, and endocrine disturbances have been added.

Seventy-six new color reproductions and 65 reproductions of radiographs have been added bringing the total number of illustrations to 543. We believe that these new illustrations, from our personal collections and from those of other oral pathologists who have generously lent their material, will enhance the value of the Atlas. The text has been rewritten wherever newer concepts and knowledge have become available. A new section, the *Diagnostic Guide,* has been added at the beginning of the Atlas. It is designed to provide a quick referral to assist the clinician in determining the name and nature of various lesions. The bibliography has been expanded to include important references concerning the diseases and lesions that have been discussed.

We believe that the fifth edition of *Colby, Kerr, and Robinson's Color Atlas of Oral Pathology* can serve as a useful source of information on oral pathology, oral medicine, and diagnosis for students and practitioners of dentistry and medicine. As a chairside reference it is designed to be a succinct source of practical information and a diagnostic guide.

Hamilton B. G. Robinson, D.D.S., M.S., D.Sc. (Hon.)
Arthur S. Miller, D.M.D., M.S.D.

Acknowledgments

The color transparencies are primarily from the University of Michigan, the Ohio State University, the University of Missouri–Kansas City, the United States Navy, and from our personal collections. The following illustrations came from other individuals and institutions and we gratefully acknowledge their contributions: American Dental Association (118, *bottom*); American Medical Association (160, *bottom*); Armed Forces Institute of Pathology (154, *center*, and 174, *top*); Drs. Paul E. Boyle and N. Dinnerman (54, *top*); Dr. Jerry Bouquot (103, *top*); Dr. George Blozis (148, *top*, 151, *top*, and 164, *top*); Dr. Joseph Calderazzo (128, *center*); Dr. W. J. Carter (89, *bottom*); Dr. D. L. Catena and W. B. Saunders Co. © 1974 (41, *center*, and 42, *bottom*); Dr. S.-Y. Chen (88, *center*, and 128, *bottom*); Dr. J. E. Fantasia (33, *top*, 86, *center*, 163, *center*, and 163, *bottom*); Dr. P. A. Farber and Springer–Verlag N.Y., Inc. © 1987 (86, *top*, and 98, *bottom*); Dr. Arnold Freedman (123, *top*); Dr. Michael Glick (122, *bottom*); Drs. H. Goldberg and Paul Goldhaber (134, *bottom*); Drs. James Hamner III and A. S. Ketchum and J. B. Lippincott Co., *Cancer* 23:1136 © 1969 (128, *top*); Drs. Robert Harwick and J. E. Fantasia (121, *top*, and 121, *bottom*); Dr. H. T. Hartsook (47, *top*); Dr. Stanley Hazen (78, *top*); Dr. H. L. Hubinger, (24, *center*); Dr. E. T. Lally (176, *top*); Dr. David Litwack (35, *center*, 35, *bottom*, and 155, *top*); Dr. César López (39, *bottom*); Drs. H. B. Marble and Henry H. Scofield (167, *bottom*); Dr. M. W. McCrea and C.V. Mosby Co., *Oral Surg, Oral Med, Oral Pathol* 25:590 © 1968 (135, *center*); Dr. Raymond Melrose (100, *top*); Memorial Hospital, New York City (129, *top*, 129, *center*, 137, *top*, 150, *top*, 152, *top*, 161, *top*, 168, *center*, 169, *top*, 173, *top*, and 175, *top*); Drs. C. S. Miller, R. M. Craig, Jr., and Ralph Correll and American Dental Association, *J Am Dent Assoc* 117:345 © 1988 (139, *center*); Drs. Moore and L. H. Jorsted (90, *top*); Dr. S. A. Passo (62, *bottom*); Dr. Nicholas Prusack (160, *center*); Dr. Peter Pullon (27, *center*, 31, *bottom*, 49, *center*, and 67, *center*); Dr. Peter Pullon and American Medical Association, *Arch Otolaryngol* 103:349 © 1977 (160, *bottom*); Drs. Peter Pullon and Marshall Manne (79, *bottom*); Dr. Peter Pullon and W. B. Saunders Co © 1974 (144, *top*); Dr. Peter Quinn (122, *top*); Dr. Peter J. Robinson (88, *bottom*); Dr. Henry H. Scofield (54, *center*); Dr. W. M. Searcy, Jr. (36, *top*); Dr. A. E. Seyler (38, *center*); Drs. Lauri Staretz, Ralph Correll and Thomas Schott and the American Dental Association, *J Am Dent Assoc* 117:185 © 1988 (88, *top*); Dr. Samuel Seltzer and Lea & Febiger © 1988 (58, *center*); Dr. Ray T. Stewart and C. V. Mosby Co, *Oral Surg* 46:831–836 © 1978 (48, *bottom*); Dr. R. C. Weiss (76, *bottom*); Dr. H. A. Zander (63, *center* and *bottom*). The sketches on pages 12 and 13 were prepared by Mrs. Warren Hedman. Numerous other individuals contributed in many ways to this Atlas. While they are not acknowledged individually the authors hope they will realize that their assistance was deeply appreciated. We also wish to recognize our wives, Kitty R. and Kathy M., for their understanding and patience.

HBGR and *ASM*

Contents

III
Diseases of the Teeth and Supporting Structures   51

IV
Diseases of the Oral Soft Tissues   85

V
Non-neoplastic Conditions of the Jaw Bones   **125**

VI
Genetic, Metabolic, and Endocrine Disturbances   **133**

VII
Neoplasms   **143**

Diagnostic Guide

Diseases and lesions are listed in accordance with their clinical or radiographic appearance to serve the clinician who is seeking to identify an entity observed in a patient. The page number is given for each entity appearing in the Atlas. Lesions of the teeth are listed in Chapter III.

Radiolucencies

Radiopacities

Cysts

Vesicles, Blisters, Bullae

Ulcers

Pigmentations

Red Lesions

White Lesions

Some lesions may be red in one phase and white in another, and some may show areas of redness and whiteness simultaneously.

Swellings and Enlargements

Colby, Kerr, and Robinson's
Color Atlas of
Oral Pathology

I Histology and Embryology

INTRODUCTION

In order to recognize and understand the abnormal it is necessary to have an understanding of the normal. It is important to know the typical gross and microscopic appearance of various tissues and to be familiar with normal development. Many individuals become frustrated in the study of pathology because they believe that their knowledge of histology and embryology is inadequate. While thorough knowledge in these two areas is of great advantage, one may begin to develop an understanding of disease adequate for the intelligent practice of dentistry on the basis of a reasonably limited background. The graduate of the modern dental school has been taught the basic information, and this section of the Atlas is designed to aid in reviewing that knowledge. It has not been planned as a replacement for standard textbooks in histology and embryology but only to present the essential information concerning the recognition of tissues and the development of the head and the neck that one should have in order to approach the study of pathology intelligently.

Before examining histopathologic material, it is necessary to be able to identify microscopically the following: skin and cutaneous appendages, oral and respiratory mucous membrane, salivary gland tissue, skeletal muscle, fibrous connective tissue, nerve tissue, cartilage, bone, enamel, dentin, cementum, pulp, and the various inflammatory cells.

Rather than trying to memorize the appearance of a given cell, tissue, or organ, one should learn the identifying characteristics of the various structures. Dependence on color to identify histologic entities is a bad practice.

In examining a tissue section, it is advisable to look at it first with the naked eye or a reversed eyepiece to learn the general characteristics of the section. When it is placed under the microscope, it should be studied first under low magnification (approximately ×30). At this magnification it is possible to determine the natural and artificial margins, the relation of one tissue to another, and any regions in which tissues vary from the normal. Areas that appear to be abnormal under low power should be examined further at a magnification of 100 or 200. Occasionally, it is necessary to investigate regional cellular detail with a magnification of 500. Oil immersion need be used only when searching for microorganisms. Some cells look nearly alike when viewed under very high power, and it is possible to identify them only by switching to a lower power and determining their arrangement and their relation to other structures. Most histopathologic material may be evaluated without resorting to a magnification higher than 100; it is a common error for those not familiar with tissue microscopy to make too great a use of the higher magnifications.

Electron microscopy adds another dimension to the study of cellular detail. However, it requires the use of special equipment that may not be available to the practicing dentist or physician.

At the molecular level of pathology immunologic technics are utilized. These do not lend themselves to illustration in this Atlas but are mentioned whenever pertinent in the text.

To learn the many details of the development of the head and neck requires concentrated and specialized study. For the practice of dentistry and the general understanding of oral pathology, it only is necessary to have a fairly detailed knowledge of tooth development and an understanding of the development of the tongue, palate, jaws, and face.

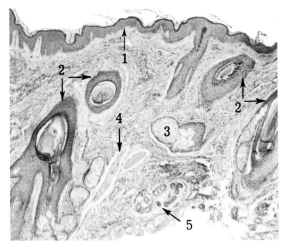

Skin ×35

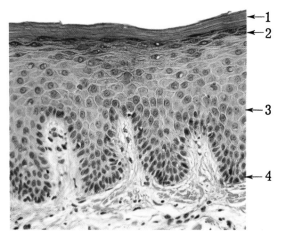

Stratified Squamous Epithelium ×220

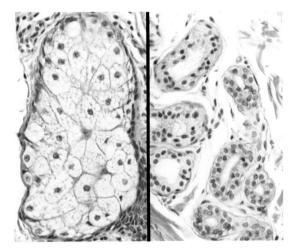

Sebaceous Gland ×200 *Sweat Gland* ×200

HISTOLOGY

Skin

(Top) The skin consists of epidermis (1), which is stratified squamous epithelium, and dermis, which is mainly connective tissue. The dermis supports the secondary skin structures, or cutaneous appendages: hair follicles (2), sebaceous glands (3), arrector pili muscles (4), and sweat glands (5).

(Center) Stratified squamous epithelium is composed of three main layers: stratum germinativum, stratum granulosum, and stratum corneum. Stratum germinativum may be subdivided into the basal layer and the prickle cell layer. The basal cell layer (4) consists of a single row of dark-staining columnar cells that are perpendicular to the dermoepidermal junction. The prickle cell layer, or stratum spinosum (3), is composed of several rows of polyhedral cells that connect with each other by desmosomes. Stratum granulosum (2) usually consists of two layers of flattened cells that contain dark-blue-staining keratohyalin granules. The stratum corneum, or horny layer (1), is made up of densely packed cells filled with keratin. The fingerlike processes of epithelium extending into the dermis are *rete pegs*. The connective tissue between two rete pegs is called a *dermal papilla*. The following terms refer to abnormalities of epithelium: *acanthosis*—hyperplasia of the prickle cell layer; *pseudoepitheliomatous hyperplasia*—benign overgrowth resembling carcinoma; *hyperorthokeratosis*—thickening of stratum corneum; *hyperparakeratosis*—retention of nuclei in cells of the stratum corneum.

(Bottom) The sebaceous gland (*left*) is composed of large polyhedral cells having small, centrally placed nuclei and abundant, light-staining, vacuolated cytoplasm. The secretion, sebum, which usually is released into a hair follicle, becomes available when the individual cells rupture. The destroyed cells are replaced from the layer of germinal epithelial cells that surround the gland. Sweat glands (*right*) are coiled structures, but they appear in microscopic sections as nests of small cut tubules, each lined by cuboidal cells. At the periphery of the tubules a few spindle-shaped myoepithelial cells may be seen.

Mucous Membrane

Oral mucous membrane differs from skin mainly in lacking secondary skin structures in the lamina propria, which is subepithelial connective tissue. Oral epithelium usually is thicker than epidermis with longer rete pegs. Most of the oral mucosa has a keratinized surface layer, although in some individuals only parakeratosis is evident. Protected areas, such as the undersurface of the tongue and the floor of the mouth, are not keratinized. A well-developed horny layer on the oral mucosa is demonstrated in the center picture on the opposite page. This photomicrograph, used to illustrate the layers of stratified squamous epithelium, is of a section from the palate.

(Top)   This illustration demonstrates the transition zone between skin and mucous membrane on the lower lip. At the far left is an abrupt termination of the hair follicles and sebaceous glands. Above this point is the vermilion border of the lip, and below it is skin. The rete pegs extend progressively deeper into the corium as the oral cavity is approached.

(Center)   Low- and high-power photomicrographs of the dentogingival junction on the lingual surface of a molar. Both the free and attached portions of the gingiva have long rete pegs that gradually diminish in size away from the free gingival margin. In higher magnification the dentogingival junction may be identified by the pale-staining cells. These, which have been separated from the cementum in preparation of the section, are derived from outer enamel epithelium. The base of the gingival crevice is at the coronal end of the dentogingival junction. The sulcus epithelium is not cornified but the external gingiva may be fairly heavily cornified.

(Bottom)   The nasal cavity proper and the paranasal sinuses (frontal, sphenoid, maxillary and ethmoid) are lined by pseudostratified ciliated columnar (respiratory) epithelium. This epithelium appears to be stratified because the nuclei are at different levels in the cells. The epithelium illustrated is from the maxillary sinus.

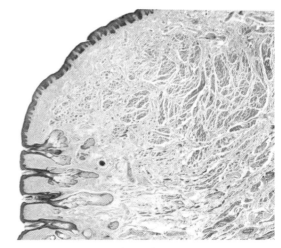

Mucocutaneous Junction, Lip   × 14

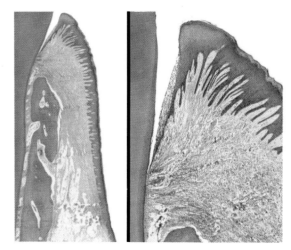

Gingiva   Left × 9, Right × 40

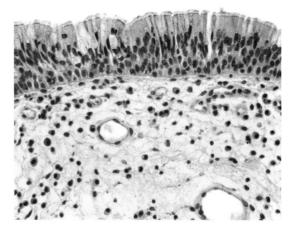

Pseudostratified Ciliated Columnar Epithelium
× 220

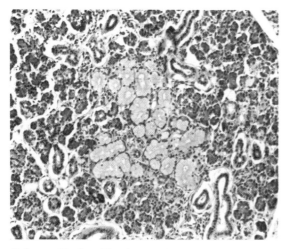

Submandibular Gland   × 60

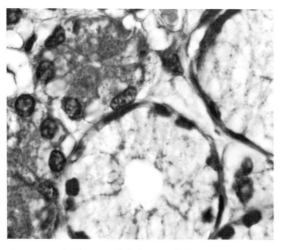

Serous and Mucous Acini   × 750

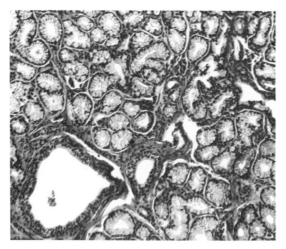

Minor Salivary Gland   × 100

Salivary Glands

The major salivary glands are composed of serous and mucous cells in the following proportions: parotid—almost pure serous; submandibular—almost 80% serous, sublingual—usually more mucous than serous, but at least half mucous. The minor salivary glands (located nearly everywhere in the oral mucosa but especially in the lips, palate, buccal mucosa, and tongue) are predominantly mucous except for the serous glands of von Ebner that open into the groove around each vallate papilla.

(Top)   Salivary gland tissue composed mainly of serous acini, which at this magnification appear as groups of dark-staining cells. The light-staining units in the center of the field are mucous acini. The structures with the large lumina are ducts.

(Center)   A mucous acinus (bottom of picture) is composed of triangular-appearing cells that are arranged in a circle, forming a distinct lumen. The nuclei of these cells are compressed against the basement membrane, and the cytoplasm is nearly colorless when stained with hematoxylin and eosin. A serous acinus (upper left) differs from the mucous type in that the nuclei of the individual cells are spherical, larger, and not compressed against the basement membrane, though they are situated near it. The cytoplasm of serous cells contains dark-blue-staining zymogen granules. Serous acini tend to be smaller than the mucous variety, and their lumina are rarely visible. A mixed acinus usually consists of a mucous unit partially surrounded by a cap of serous cells (serous demilune).

(Bottom)   In this section of salivary gland tissue, which is from the lip, the acini are all of the mucous type. Ducts are evident near the lower border. The duct system varies in the different salivary glands, but, in general, the peripheral ducts adjacent to the lobules of the gland are small and lined by a single row of short epithelial cells. Approaching the surface, the ducts become larger and are lined by taller cells. Close to the surface there is often a double row of cells. Finally, the last portion of the duct is lined by squamous epithelium from the oral cavity.

Tongue

(Top) Histologic section through the tip of the tongue, demonstrating papillated dorsal surface and relatively smooth undersurface. The red-staining material that makes up the bulk of the tongue is voluntary muscle running in all directions. This complex musculature is peculiar to the tongue. The light-blue-staining areas (groups of mucous acini) constitute the anterior lingual gland.

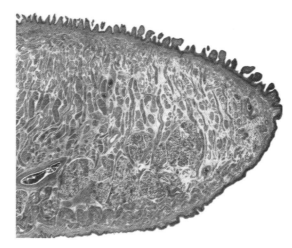

Tongue, Sagittal Section, Newborn Infant   ×11

(Center) Voluntary (skeletal) muscle fibers are extremely large, multinucleated cells composed of numerous myofibrils. The identifying features of skeletal muscle—cross striations and peripherally placed nuclei—are apparent in this photomicrograph of two longitudinally cut fibers. In cross section the fibers appear as eosinophilic islands, some of which have rounded nuclei situated just under the cell membrane.

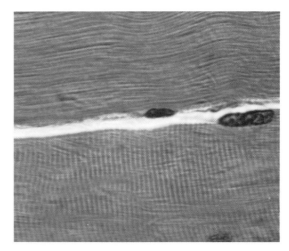

Voluntary Muscle   ×1080

(Bottom) There are three main types of lingual papillae—filiform, fungiform, and vallate (circumvallate). The filiform papillae (*upper left*) are small, conical epithelial projections with rather thick keratinized layers. The amount of keratinization of these, the most numerous of the papillae, is reflected in the degree of tongue coating. The fungiform papillae (*upper right*) are scattered among the filiform papillae, being most numerous toward the sides and tip of the tongue. They are toadstool-like projections of connective tissue covered by relatively thin layers of epithelium. Clinically, these papillae appear as small red nodules because the thin epithelium does not mask the color of the underlying vascular connective tissue. The vallate papillae (*lower*), 8 to 12 in number, are arranged in an inverted V just anterior to the root of the tongue. The apex of the V is close to the foramen cecum. Each of these papillae (see p. 26, *top,* for the gross appearance) protrudes slightly and is surrounded by a deep groove. In some individuals rudimentary foliate papillae (see p. 26, *center*), which may be associated with lymphoid nodules, appear as parallel folds of mucosa on the lateral margins of the tongue posteriorly.

Taste buds (*arrow*) are seen as intraepithelial light-staining ovoid structures. Although most common in the vallate papillae, they may also be noted in the foliate and in some of the fungiform papillae.

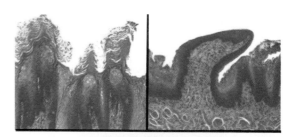

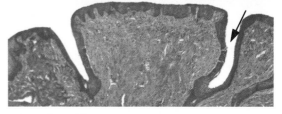

Lingual Papillae   Upper ×35, Lower ×28

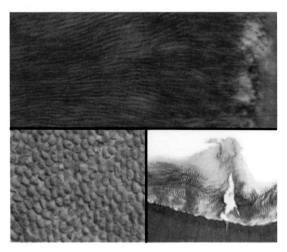

Enamel   Upper ×427, Lower Left ×513,
Lower Right ×100

Enamel

(Top)   Newly formed enamel matrix is shown in the upper photomicrograph. A small area of dentin is seen at the right. Despite decalcification of this specimen, the enamel is well preserved because at this stage of development it has not undergone much mineralization. In the ground cross section of mature enamel (*lower left*) the ends of the enamel rods, as well as the interrod substance, may be seen. The appearance of rods cut in this plane has been likened to fish scales. In the lower right photomicrograph is a decalcified section of an erupted tooth. The dentin is at the lower border, and above this is a remnant of the acid-insoluble organic enamel matrix.

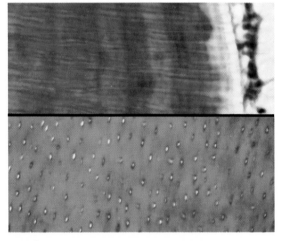

Dentin   Upper ×550, Lower ×490

Dentin

(Center)   In the upper half of the illustration, a row of odontoblasts is seen at the right. To the left of this region is a band of pale-staining predentin, and further to the left is calcified dentin. The light streaks that extend from the odontoblasts through the predentin and dentin are tubules that contain the odontoblastic process. The lower photomicrograph illustrates the dentinal tubules cut in cross section.

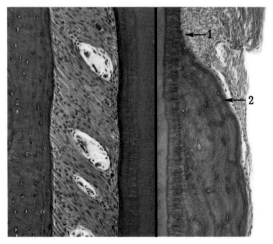

Periodontal Ligament   ×100   Cementium   ×100

Periodontal Ligament and Cementum

(Bottom)   In the center of the left photomicrograph are oblique fibers of the periodontal ligament that are attached to alveolar bone (*left*) and cementum (*right*). The oval light-staining areas, between the bundles of principal fibers, are composed of very loose connective tissue in which are nerves, blood vessels, and lymphatics. The right photomicrograph demonstrates acellular cementum (1) and cellular cementum (2). The first cementum deposited against the dentin is usually of the acellular variety. There is a slow but continuous formation of cementum throughout the life of the tooth that compensates for tooth movement and allows new fibers of the periodontal ligament to be embedded in the surface of the root.

Pulp

(Top) Cross section of the coronal pulp of a third molar from a 21-year-old patient. The pulp consists of delicate, loose connective tissue in which there are numerous blood vessels, lymph vessels, and nerves. Odontoblasts constitute the outermost portion of the pulp. In young pulp the fibroblasts, which are somewhat star-shaped, are quite numerous, but with age the pulp may become less cellular and more fibrous.

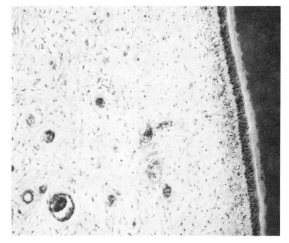

Pulp × 100

Cartilage and Bone

(Center) Hyaline cartilage (*left*) is identified easily by its lavender-staining homogeneous matrix. In the matrix are spaces that contain 1 to 4 large cells with prominent centrally placed nuclei. In the upper portion of the illustration is a dense layer of fibrous connective tissue, the perichondrium, from which appositional growth takes place. The right photomicrograph is a low-power view to demonstrate compact bone (*above*) and trabecular bone (*below*). The relatively clear spaces enclosed by the trabecular bone are composed mainly of yellow or fatty marrow. Trabecular (spongy or cancellous) bone may be changed to the compact type by the deposition of layers of new bone on the sides of the trabeculae, so that finally the marrow spaces are reduced to small channels that contain only blood vessels. Bone is not a static substance, for its architecture is constantly changing (remodeling) in accordance with functional needs.

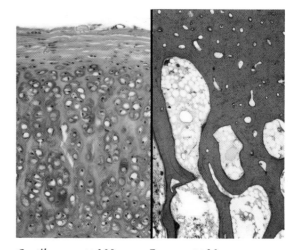

Cartilage × 100   *Bone* × 20

(Bottom) Osteoclasts are present at (1) and osteoblasts at (2) in the left photomicrograph. The osteoclasts (*upper right*) are large multinucleated cells that are associated with bone resorption. Usually they are seen in small harborlike spaces (Howship's lacunae). Osteoblasts (*lower right*) are spindle-shaped cells that secrete the organic intercellular substance of bone. Many of the osteoblasts become surrounded by this intercellular substance and remain in the bone as osteocytes. The vitality of bone is determined histologically by the presence of osteocytes.

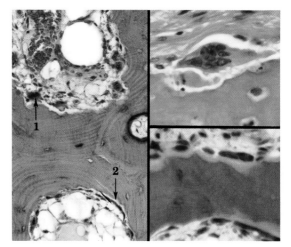

Osteoclasts and Osteoblasts   Left × 190,
Right Upper × 456, *Lower* × 380

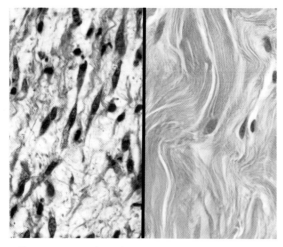

Fibrous Connective Tissue   × 448

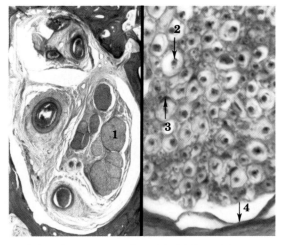

Peripheral Nerve   Left × 16, Right × 520

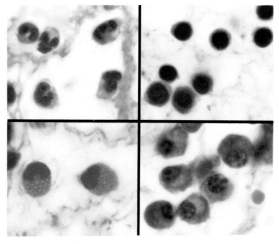

Inflammatory Cells   × 1080

Fibrous Connective Tissue

(Top)   Loose, immature connective tissue (*left*) has many young fibroblasts that have spindle-shaped nuclei and long cytoplasmic processes. Fibroblasts are responsible for the elaboration of collagen and the intercellular portion of connective tissue. It seems certain, however, that the fibers are not extensions of these cells. Dense, mature fibrous connective tissue (*right*) has only a few fibrocytes, being composed mainly of eosinophilic collagen fibers.

Peripheral Nerve

(Center)   Cross section (*left*) through posterior portion of the mandibular nerve. One of the fasciculi of the nerve (1) is enlarged in the photomicrograph at right. An axis-cylinder is seen at (2), surrounded by a clear space that, before preparation of the specimen, was occupied by myelin. At the periphery of the myelin is the neurilemma (sheath of Schwann). A nucleus of a Schwann cell is apparent at (3). A connective tissue sheath, epineurium, surrounds the several fasciculi of a nerve. The perineurium (4) envelops each individual fasciculus. Connective tissue extending into fasciculi is termed endoneurium.

Inflammatory Cells

(Bottom)   The following types of inflammatory cells, with their distingushing characteristics, are shown: Neutrophils (*upper left*)—finely granular cytoplasm staining light bluish pink; nuclei with 3 to 5 lobes. Lymphocytes (*upper right*)—varying in size; very thin rim of cytoplasm around circular deep-purple-staining nucleus. Eosinophils (*lower left*)—coarsely granular reddish cytoplasm; 1- or 2-lobed nuclei. Plasma cells (*lower right*)—eccentrically placed nuclei, having appearance of cartwheel or clock face because of clumped arrangement of chromatin; lavender cytoplasm, often pale near nucleus, producing halo-like effect. The size of these various cells may be judged by comparison with erythrocyte (7.6 μm) in lower right picture.

Inflammation is the body's response to any irritant that has the potential to injure or kill cells. Neutrophils, which are transported by the blood, are the first cells to arrive at the region of injury. They ingest bacteria and provide proteolytic enzymes that can liquify injured cells. Lymphocytes come via the blood or may migrate from lymphoid tissue in the region. They are present in all stages of inflammation but are most numerous in chronic stages. There are two lines of lymphocytes, one concerned with cell-mediated immunity (T-lymphocytes) and the other with humoral immunity (B-lymphocytes). Lymphocytes may harbor viral DNA that can be transported to other regions or reactivate disease in carriers. Large granular lymphocytes are involved in killer cell activity and form part of the body's defense against malignant cells as well as against infective agents. Plasma cells usually are prominent in chronic oral lesions, originating from small lymphocytes and synthesizing antibodies. Eosinophils probably originate in the marrow. They are slightly phagocytic and are most numerous in inflammations of an allergic nature, in parasitism, and in certain long-standing chronic processes. Macrophages, which are the second line of defense, assist the neutrophils in the ingestion and the digestion of bacteria. They phagocytize tissue debris, thus preparing the area for repair. These scavenger-type cells may be from the blood (large mononuclears) or from other tissues. Those of histogenous origin are known by various names, such as histiocytes, endothelial leukocytes, resting-wandering cells, clasmatocytes, polyblasts, and cells of the reticuloendothelial system.

(Top) Large lipid-containing macrophages are shown in the upper section. The nuclei have been pushed to one side, and the cytoplasm consists of vacuoles, the fat having been lost during processing of the specimen. Neutrophils have been engulfed by the macrophage in the lower left picture. A hemosiderin-containing macrophage is seen in the lower right section.

(Center) A foreign body giant cell (*left*) with numerous haphazardly situated nuclei; (*right*) a similar cell surrounding suture material.

(Bottom) Numerous lens-shaped slits (*left*) formerly occupied by cholesterol crystals. Enlargement (*right*) shows foreign body giant cells in close apposition to a crystal. Cholesterol crystals may be found whenever there has been tissue disintegration; they are common in walls of periodontal cysts.

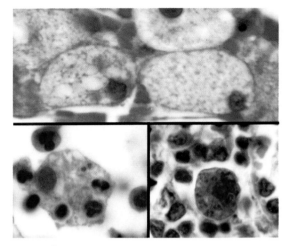

Macrophages × 1080

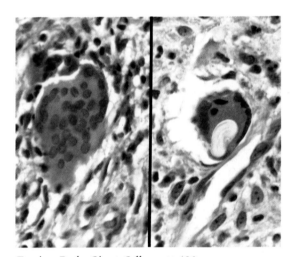

Foreign Body Giant Cells × 490

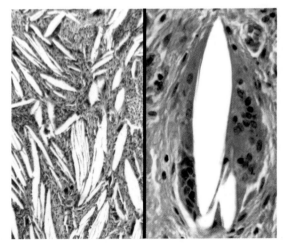

Cholesterol Slits and Foreign Body Giant Cells
Left × 62, *Right* × 387

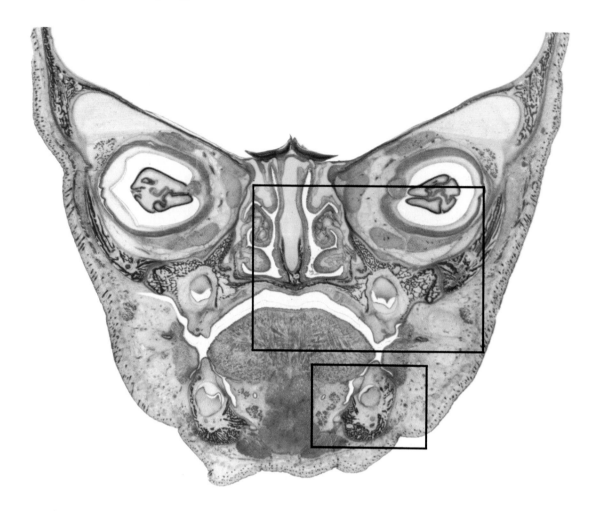

Frontal Section Through Head of Human Fetus (6 Months) in Region of Deciduous Molars   × 4

EMBRYOLOGY

Human Fetus

In the enlargements (*opposite page*) of the blocked areas shown above, the following structures are evident:

1	Developing eye
2	Optic nerve
3	Extrinsic eye muscles
4	Infraorbital nerve
5	Inferior, middle, and superior conchae
6	Respiratory epithelium
7	Nasal cavity
8	Nasal septum
9	Maxillary bone
10	Dorsal surface of tongue
11	Palatal glands
12	Developing teeth
13	Zygomatic bone (malar)
14	Parotid duct
15	Buccinator muscle
16	Tongue muscle
17	Dental lamina
18	Oral epithelium
19	Submandibular gland duct (Wharton's)
20	Sublingual gland
21	Meckel's cartilage
22	Mylohyoid muscle
23	Anterior belly of the digastric muscle
24	Bone of mandible
25	Mandibular nerve
26	Mandibular vessels
27	Platysma muscle
28	Epidermis of the face
29	Lanugo hair follicle

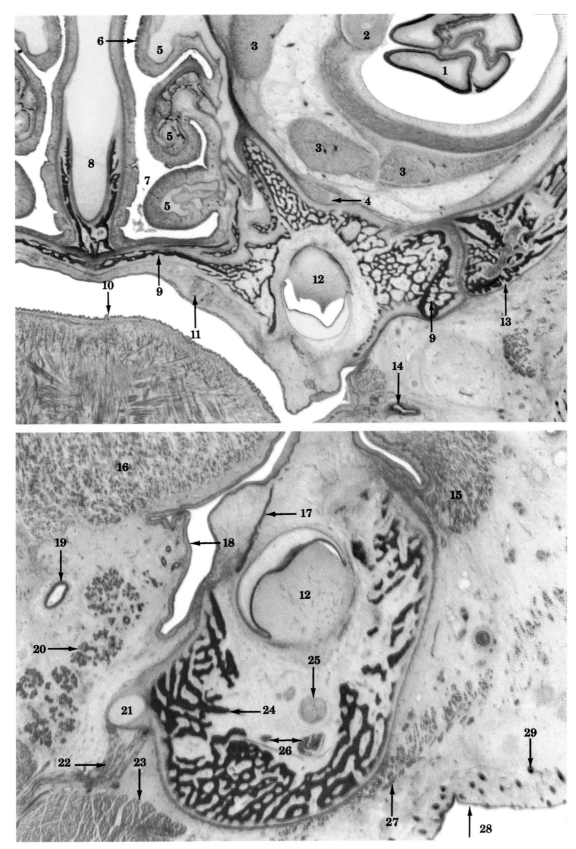

Frontal Section Through Head of Human Fetus Upper ×9.6, Lower ×20

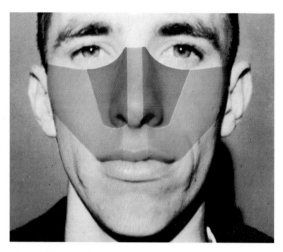

Embryonic Derivations of Various Parts of the Face

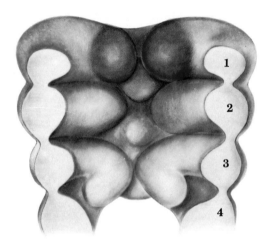

Sketch of Anterior View of Pharynx, Seen from Within Human Embryo (3 Weeks)

Development of the Face

(Top) The colors superimposed on the adult face designate areas derived from the following embryonic structures: mandibular arch (yellow), maxillary processes (blue green), medial nasal process (blue), lateral nasal processes (red).

Branchial Arches

(Center) The external depressions between the branchial bars or arches (1 through 4) are branchial clefts, while the furrows on the inside are termed pharyngeal pouches. The clefts and the external surfaces of the arches are bordered by ectodermal epithelium, while the pouches and internal surfaces of the arches (except the 1st) are bordered by endodermal epithelium. At a certain stage the epithelium of the pouches on the inside meets the epithelium of the external clefts, with no mesoderm between them. In lower animals, like the fish, this double epithelial membrane ruptures, and gill slits result, but in humans the arches merge by the process of mesenchymal tissue proliferation, which pushes the epithelia of the pouches and clefts inward and outward, finally presenting smooth inner and outer surfaces. The pouches are the origin of numerous structures, among which are the middle ear (1st pouch), palatine tonsil (2nd pouch), and parathyroid glands (3rd and 4th pouches).

Development of the Tongue

(Center) The tongue develops from the internal surfaces of the 1st, 2nd, and 3rd branchial arches by 4 nodular swellings. The anterior portion, or body, is formed from the 1st arch by 2 lateral prominences (red) and 1 medial prominence, the tuberculum impar (blue). The posterior portion, or root, is formed from the copula, which is the nodule seen just below the blue-colored tuberculum impar.

(Bottom) The 3 prominences forming the anterior part of the tongue are about equal in size at this stage. As development progresses, the tuberculum impar (blue) stops growing and partially degenerates, allowing the 2 lateral prominences (red) to grow over it and meet in the midline.

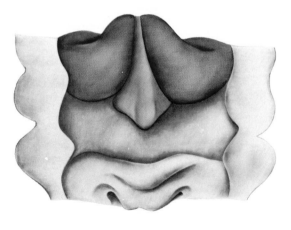

Developing Tongue (5 Weeks)

(Top)   The two lateral halves of the tongue have now united (line of fusion shown in black). The diamond-shaped area (broken blue line) represents the final position of the tuberculum impar beneath the surface of the tongue. Small circle indicates the foramen cecum. (This picture and the three on p. 12 modified after Sicher and Tandler.)

Thyroglossal Duct

The thyroid gland develops from an epithelium-lined tube (thyroglossal duct) that arises from an area between the copula and the tuberculum impar. (See center picture, opposite page.) This tube grows downward through the tongue and through a region that later will become hyoid bone to a point in the midline of the neck, where the thyroid gland is formed from it. After forming the thyroid gland the duct should involute. Its point of origin on the tongue is indicated permanently by an enlarged pit, the foramen cecum. (See top picture.)

(Center)   Low-power photomicrograph (*left*) illustrates that at this stage of development the embryo still has a marked dorsal convexity, with the large head curved forward and the short mandible lying tight against the chest. A small channel may be seen extending into the primitive oral cavity, which at this stage is occupied mostly by the tongue. Just below the oral opening is the heart. The large organ near the bottom of the picture is the liver. Enlargement (*right*) of blocked area (*left*) shows base of tongue, oral cavity, pharynx, esophagus, and trachea. The thyroglossal duct can be seen extending from the foramen cecum (*arrow*) through the tongue to a region just in front of the developing hyoid bone. At this age the duct should begin to involute.

(Bottom)   Frontal section through tongue in region of the foramen cecum. A persistent thyroglossal duct, lined by stratified squamous epithelium, extends almost to the hyoid bone. Nonlingual remnants of such a duct usually consist of pseudostratified columnar epithelium. Thyroglossal duct (tract) cysts may arise from these embryonal remnants (see page 22).

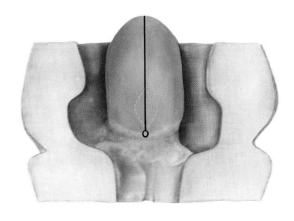

Sketch of Anterior Part of Tongue, Human Embryo (6 Weeks)

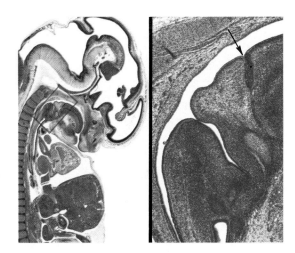

Human Embryo (7 Weeks), Sagittal Section Left × 7, Right × 40

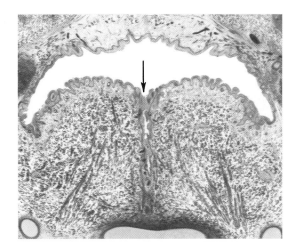

Persistent Thyroglossal Duct, Human Fetus (5 Months)   × 14

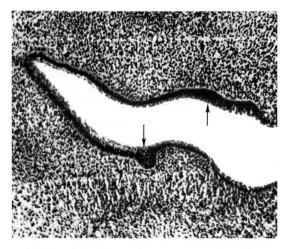

Initiation of Tooth Development, Frontal Section, Human Embryo (6 Weeks)   × 40

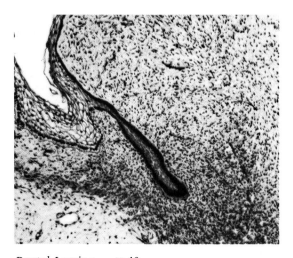

Dental Lamina   × 40

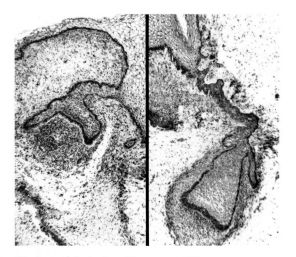

Early and Late Cap Stages   × 25

Tooth Development

Tooth development is composed of the following physiologic processes: stimulation of certain cells to multiply (initiation and proliferation); establishment of tooth pattern (morphodifferentiation); differentiation of cells to perform special functions (histodifferentiation); formation of dentin and enamel matrix (apposition); influx of mineral salts and their subsequent crystallization (calcification and maturation); emergence of the crown into the oral cavity (eruption).

(Top)   Initiation. Human tooth development begins, usually between the 35th and 42nd days *in utero*, by a thickening of the primitive oral epithelium (*arrows*) in areas that are destined to become the maxillary and mandibular ridges. This epithelial thickening, which extends along the length of both jaws, is termed the *dental lamina*.

(Center)   Proliferation. In 10 locations along each jaw the dental lamina proliferates into the primitive connective tissue. One of these extensions is shown. Eventually, cells of this epithelial structure will form the enamel portion of the tooth, while cells derived from the surrounding mesenchymal tissue will form dentin, pulp, cementum, periodontal ligament, and alveolar bone.

(Bottom)   Morphodifferentiation. Each proliferating epithelial extension becomes large at the end, developing a concave lower surface that somewhat resembles a cap (*left*). The mesenchymal tissue within the confines of the cap changes its character by becoming quite cellular. Eventually, this portion of connective tissue will be the dental pulp. As development of the primary tooth progresses (*right*), the epithelial cells at the lower portion of the enamel organ become columnar (inner enamel epithelium), while the remaining peripheral cells are cuboidal (outer enamel epithelium). The epithelial cells in the central portion of the enamel organ begin to separate, initiating the formation of the stellate reticulum. The mesodermal tissue surrounding the whole structure becomes condensed, forming the connective tissue follicle, or dental sac. The epithelial extension seen near the right border of the picture is the primordium of a succedaneous tooth which will go through the same developmental processes as did the primary tooth.

(Top) At this stage of development the dental lamina is just beginning to disintegrate. The inner enamel epithelium (ameloblastic layer) has become stabilized, thus establishing the future dentino-enamel junction, which reflects the ultimate shape of the tooth (morphodifferentiation and histodifferentiation). Disturbances during these stages of tooth development may result in dental anomalies (see pp. 35–49).

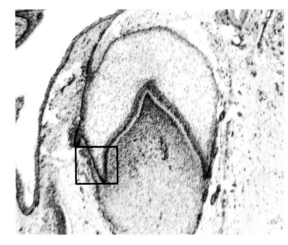

Advanced Bell Stage   × 40

(Center) In an enlargement of the blocked area from above, the outer enamel epithelium (1) meets the inner enamel epithelum (4) to form the cervical loop, the tip of which proliferates apically to become Hertwig's sheath after the enamel is fully apposed (see p. 16 *center*). The stellate reticulum (2) resembles young loose connective tissue but actually is composed of star-shaped epithelial cells that, except for fine threadlike connections, are widely separated from each other by a mucoid substance. The stratum intermedium (3) consists of a few rows of cells that are essential for the actual deposition of enamel matrix by ameloblasts. The dental papilla is identified at (5).

(Bottom) High-power view (*right*), from side of enamel organ, identifies the stellate reticulum (1), stratum intermedium (2), ameloblasts (3), odontoblasts (4), and dental papilla (5). The ameloblasts at the bottom of the low-power photomicrograph (*left*) have large, centrally placed nuclei, and adjacent to them is a clear, cell-free area in the dental papilla. The ameloblasts near the middle of the picture have elongated at the expense of the clear area, and their nuclei are situated at the stratum intermedium end. These ameloblasts have influenced cells of the dental papilla to become odontoblasts, some of which have already participated in the formation of dentin (orange). After dentin is formed, the ameloblasts receive their nutrient supply from the dental sac, for their former source (the dental papilla) is blocked by dentin. At the upper border (*left*) the enamel matrix appears as a thin black line between the ameloblasts and the dentin. Connective tissue cells do not differentiate into odontoblasts without the organizing influence of the inner enamel epithelium, and the ameloblasts do not commence amelogenesis until laying down of dentin has begun.

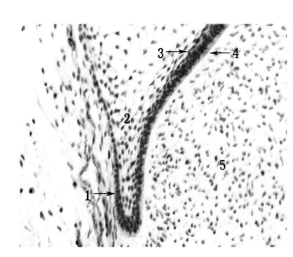

Cervical Loop   × 100

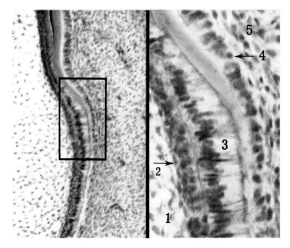

Cell Changes Associated with Early Dentin and Enamel Formation   *Left* × 100, *Right* × 950

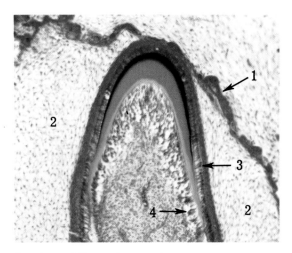

Dentin and Enamel Formation   × 100

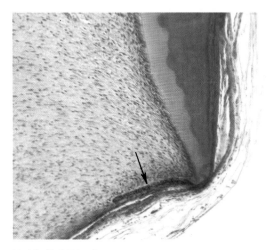

Epithelial Diaphragm   × 100

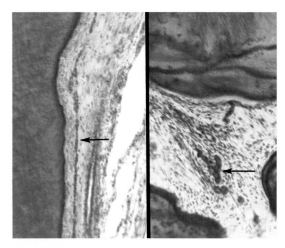

Remnants of Hertwig's Sheath
Left × 100, *Right* × 950

(Top) The incisal tip is capped by enamel matrix (black) and dentin matrix (red). The outer enamel epithelium is at (1), the stellate reticulum at (2), the ameloblastic layer at (3), and the odontoblasts at (4). Near the top of the picture the stellate reticulum has disappeared and the cells of the outer enamel epithelium are in contact with the stratum intermedium. After enamel formation is completed the stratum intermedium, outer enamel epithelium, and the ameloblastic cells (now reduced in height) fuse and persist until the tooth emerges into the oral cavity. As the tooth approaches the surface, the reduced enamel epithelium and the oral epithelium fuse. After eruption the epithelium attached to the tooth surface forms the dentogingival junction. The transformation of enamel matrix into hard enamel begins with the influx of minerals in an organic state. The process whereby the proper crystalline structure of the enamel is gradually developed by the conversion of these minerals to an inorganic form is termed *maturation.*

(Center) Hertwig's sheath, which consists of inner and outer enamel epithelium, is responsible for root shape and for initiating the formation of root dentin. This double row of epithelial cells proliferates apically from the future cementoenamel junction and abruptly turns inward to form the epithelial diaphragm *(arrow).* The inner enamel epithelium induces adjacent pulpal cells to become odontoblasts, and dentinogenesis begins. As root dentin is formed, the tooth migrates coronally, allowing the continuously proliferating epithelial diaphragm to remain in its original relation.

(Bottom) Immediately after root dentin begins to form in any given area, connective tissue of the dental sac grows inward and perforates Hertwig's sheath, obliterating much of it. The dental sac becomes the periodontal ligament, and its innermost cells form cementum while its outermost cells form the alveolar bone. Remnants of Hertwig's sheath (cell rests of Malassez) are seen near the lateral surface of a root *(left, arrow)* and in periapical tissue *(right, arrow).* Varying amounts of cell rests are present in all periodontal ligaments and may be sources of odontogenic cysts and tumors.

II Developmental Disturbances

INTRODUCTION

Developmental disturbances may be classified in order of increasing severity as variations, anomalies, malformations, and monstrosities. Variations are quite minor deviations from normal (*e.g.*, large oral orifice); anomalies are more severe but do not interfere with function (*e.g.*, enamel hypoplasia, peg laterals); malformations are even more severe and interfere with function (*e.g.*, cleft lip); and monstrosities are extreme deviations which severely interfere with function (*e.g.*, agnathia, dicephalus).

Some abnormalities result largely from intrinsic factors (heredity, metabolic dysfunction, mutations); others largely from extrinsic factors (physical or chemical agents, living agents, nutritional deficiency, stress). In some instances both intrinsic and extrinsic factors play a part.

Certain developmental disturbances are apparent at birth (congenital); others, though determined before birth, may not be evident until later. Some noncongenital developmental defects result entirely from postnatal environmental influences on structures still developing.

Many developmental defects of the head-and-neck region result from failure of embryonic processes to unite properly. These failures may cause clefts of the face, the lips, the alveolus, or the hard or soft palate. Incomplete union of the maxillary and mandibular processes produces a very large oral orifice (macrostomia), while union extending too far anteriorly causes a small oral opening (microstomia). If the two lateral halves of the tongue fail to unite anteriorly, a bifid tongue results.

Because much of the intricate development of the head-and-neck region involves epithelium, many opportunities are afforded for the enclavement of epithelial cells. These residual epithelial cells then become potential sources of cysts (closed pathologic epithelium-lined spaces), sinuses (pathologic epithelium-lined spaces opening onto a body surface or into a natural cavity), and fistulae (abnormal epithelium-lined tracts opening upon two surfaces). Epithelium trapped during the uniting of embryonic processes either by faulty merging or by faulty fusion may form branchial cleft, epidermoid, dermoid, globulomaxillary, or median palatine cysts. Incomplete involution of Hertwig's sheath, the dental lamina, the nasopalatine ducts, or the thyroglossal duct may leave epithelium to form cysts in the respective regions. Everyone has some residual epithelium in the head-and-neck region, but only a few develop cysts from it, for cyst formation is dependent upon proliferation of the residual epithelium. Inflammation is definitely known to stimulate epithelium to form periodontal cysts, but for most other cysts the exciting cause seldom is apparent.

Auricular tags, Fordyce spots, lingual thyroid, and enamel pearls are examples of normal tissues developing in abnormal sites.

Primordial cysts form because of regressive changes in tooth buds. The formation of dentigerous cysts occurs at a later stage of odontogenesis. Failure of the tuberculum impar to involute may be, in part, the cause of median rhomboid glossitis.

Hygroma, tori, macroglossia, hypercementosis, supernumerary teeth, and some of the odontomas are examples of excessive growth.

Among the disturbances resulting from underdevelopment are micrognathia, dwarfed roots, microdontia, anodontia, enamel hypoplasia, and enamel hypocalcification.

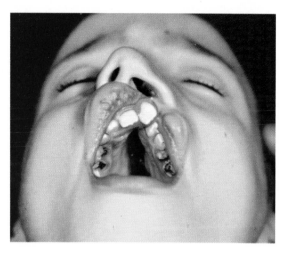

Unilateral Cleft Lip and Cleft Palate

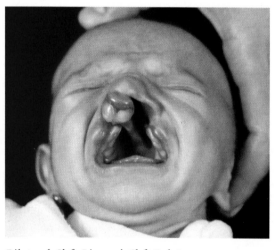

Bilateral Cleft Lip and Cleft Palate

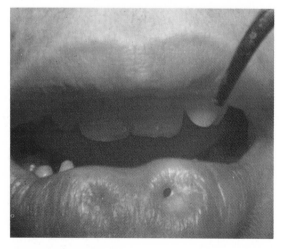

Congenital Lip Pits

CLEFTS OF THE LIP AND THE PALATE

Clefts of the lip and palate are often genetic in origin. Some degree of these disturbances has been reported as occurring once in every 800 births. Clefts of the upper lip are either unilateral or bilateral, midline clefts appearing rarely in the lower lip. These malformations are due to failure of epithelium of the parts to degenerate; hence the underlying mesenchymal tissue on either side cannot unite. Clefts may be limited to the lips (cheiloschisis), the alveolus (gnathoschisis), the soft palate (staphyloschisis), or the hard and soft palate (staphylo-uranoschisis), or may present various combinations involving these structures. Extrinsic factors such as nutritional disturbances, infectious agents, and drugs have been shown, through animal experiments, to contribute to formation of clefts.

(Top)   The unilateral cleft of the lip (cheiloschisis) and the alveolar process (gnathoschisis) is due to failure of the median palatine and the left and right maxillary processes to unite. The left and right lateral palatine processes have not met or united in the midline, resulting in cleft palate (staphylo-uranoschisis).

(Center)   An extensive bilateral cleft of lip and jaw combined with a midpalatine cleft caused by failure of development of palatine processes. The globular mass is the premaxilla, which developed from the median nasal process but did not fuse with the maxillary processes.

CONGENITAL LIP PITS

(Bottom)   Congenital pits may be found as paired, paramedian structures, often exuding mucin, on the vermilion of the lower lip. Their formation may be related to failure of the bilateral grooves on the mandibular arch to fuse during early development. The pits may be an isolated finding or may be associated with cleft lip or cleft palate. Hyperplasia of the surrounding mucosa usually results in elevation of the tissue, as seen in this example.

MICROGNATHIA (BRACHYGNATHIA) AND PIERRE ROBIN SYNDROME

(Top) An example of acquired micrognathia; the heads of the condyles were damaged during forceps delivery. The growth centers for the mandible are the hyaline cartilage in the condylar heads, and injury to these areas with or without ankylosis results in cessation of development. In severe congenital micrognathia the infant may experience respiratory distress from glossoptosis and from having the tongue caught in a cleft palate (Robin, Pierre Robin syndrome). Inability to masticate, extensive speech defects, periodontal disease, and psychologic maladjustment are complications of acquired as well as congenital micrognathia.

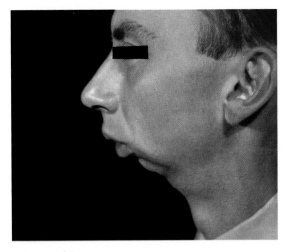

Micrognathia

HEMIATROPHY

In hemiatrophy one half of the face or the head or an entire side of the body may diminish in size. The atrophy, usually of neurogenic origin, is progressive, and the region previously of normal size becomes smaller. It should not be confused with other facial asymmetries due to unilateral underdevelopment (hypoplasia) or unilateral overdevelopment (hyperplasia).

(Center) A few years previously this individual's face was of normal contour. Now the entire right side is flattened, and the eye is deeply set. Maxillary, mandibular, and zygomatic bones as well as the facial and masticatory muscles show evidence of atrophy unilaterally. Blocking out the right or left sides of the face in this picture will show the striking differences between the normal and the atrophic appearances.

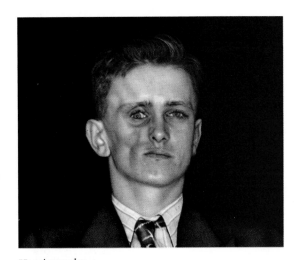

Hemiatrophy

CYSTIC HYGROMA

(Bottom) This cystic hygroma (hygroma colli congenitum) extends bilaterally. This anomaly may be present at birth but may not develop noticeably until several months thereafter. Occasionally it may be of such size that swallowing and breathing are impaired. This lesion, which is a cystic type of lymphangioma, consists of numerous large, lymph-filled, noncommunicating spaces lined by endothelium. The tumor is produced by growth, dilatation, and coalescence of embryonic lymph sacs in the neck; in some instances it extends into the mediastinum. There often is an association with congenital lymphangiomas of the tongue (see p. 151).

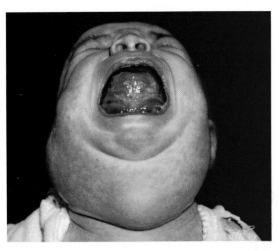

Cystic Hygroma

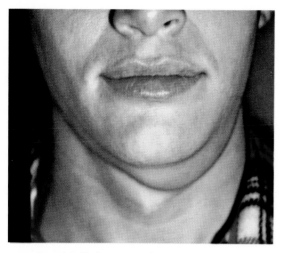

Lymphoepithelial Cyst, Neck

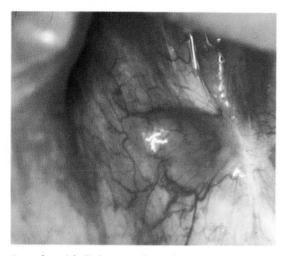

Lymphoepithelial Cyst, Floor of Mouth

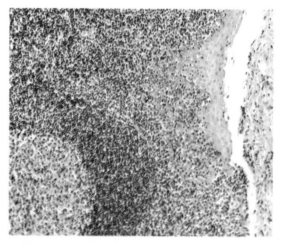

Lymphoepithelial Cyst, Floor of Mouth   × 100

LYMPHOEPITHELIAL CYST

(Top)   Lymphoepithelial (branchial arch) cyst appears as a painless, fluctuant swelling, either on the lateral aspect of the neck or in the floor of the mouth. It is never in the midline. This developmental anomaly probably originates from epithelium that is entrapped in lymph nodes. The epithelium is believed to originate from embryonic branchial arches (see p. 12) or from salivary gland epithelium. The cysts are usually lined by stratified squamous epithelium and rarely by pseudo-stratified ciliated columnar epithelium. The walls contain lymphoid tissue with germinal centers. On palpation these movable cysts vary from firm to flabby. Lymphoepithelial cysts have been termed *oral tonsils* and *tonsillocysts* because of their resemblance to tonsillar crypts. (See also p. 26). Differential diagnosis should include malignant lymphoma, salivary gland neoplasm, inflamed lymph nodes, carotid body tumor, and metastatic tumors to lymph nodes.

(Center)   A lymphoepithelial cyst in the floor of the mouth. Typically, these cysts appear in the anterior region as moderate-sized nodules. Clinically, they resemble mucoceles or lipomas, from which they should be differentiated through microscopic examination.

(Bottom)   Photomicrograph of area from cyst wall of lymphoepithelial cyst showing lining and contents. The cleft at the right is the lumen of the cyst. The rounded area at the lower left is the germinal center of the lymphoid tissue. In most cases the cyst lumen contains desquamated epithelial cells. A few will contain keratin material. The epithelium may be derived from ectopic glandular epithelium that undergoes cystic change or from crypt epithelium in continuity with surface epithelium.

EPIDERMOID CYST

Epidermoid and dermoid cysts appear similar clinically but can be differentiated histologically. When these cysts occur in the oral cavity they usually appear in the anterior portion of the floor of the mouth although they may be seen in other locations as a result of traumatic implantation (epidermal implantation cysts) or embryonic remnants. Those in the floor of the mouth may be mistaken for ranulas although the former cysts usually have thicker walls.

(Top) This epidermoid cyst in a young man measured approximately $3 \times 3 \times 4.5$ cm. It was neither tender nor painful, but was slightly fluctuant and movable. It was identified as an epidermoid cyst histologically.

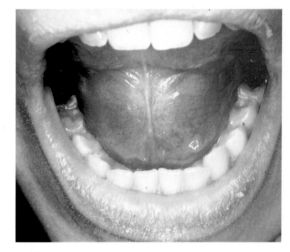

Epidermoid Cyst

(Center) The lower half of the photomicrograph shows a portion of a cyst filled with keratin and lined by flattened stratified squamous epithelium. This is an epidermoid cyst because no cutaneous appendages are present in the cyst wall. Like the dermoid cyst, this type may originate from epithelial remnants or from implanted epithelium. The cyst illustrated was removed from the vermilion portion of the lower lip, just lateral to the midline. In one stage of the development of the lower lip there are three furrows, one in the midline and one on each side of it. This cyst probably developed from misplaced islands of epithelium when one of these lateral furrows was obliterated. Paramedian lip pits may have the same origin.

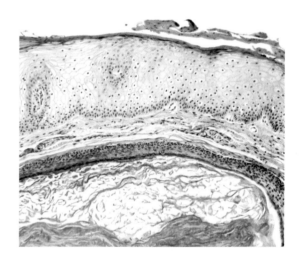

Epidermoid Cyst $\times 100$

DERMOID CYST

(Bottom) A dermoid cyst is lined by stratified squamous epithelium and has in its wall one or more skin appendages (sebaceous glands, sweat glands, hair follicles). Dermoid cysts occasionally appear below the mylohyoid muscles as extraoral swellings resembling thyroglossal duct cysts.

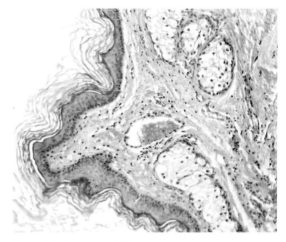

Dermoid Cyst $\times 100$

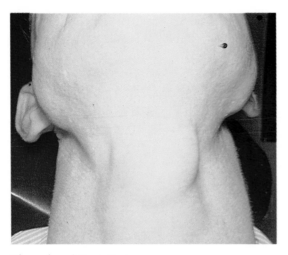

Thyroglossal Duct Cyst

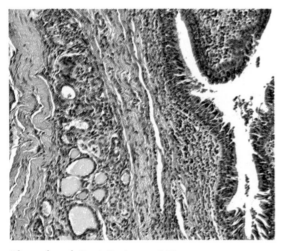

Thyroglossal Duct Cyst   × 100

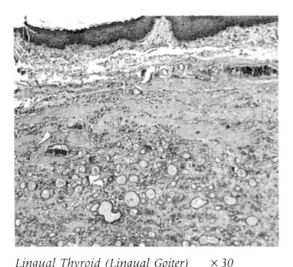

Lingual Thyroid (Lingual Goiter)   × 30

THYROGLOSSAL DUCT CYST

The thyroglossal duct (see p. 13) is an epithelium-lined tube that originates on the anterior surface of the primitive pharynx at a point between the sites of origin of the anterior and the posterior parts of the tongue. This duct during its transitory existence grows down through the tongue and the hyoid bone area to a predetermined point in the anterior aspect of the neck, where it bifurcates to form the thyroid gland. After its function is performed, it should involute, but portions of it may persist and give rise to cysts or sinuses. Because residual cells from the upper third of the duct tend to develop into stratified squamous epithelium and those from the remainder into pseudostratified columnar epithelium, the resultant cysts may be lined by either or both types.

(Top)   This large, fluctuant midline swelling is typical of the thyroglossal duct cyst in the neck. It should be differentiated from dermoid or epidermoid cysts, goiter, and thyroid neoplasm. Such cysts can occur at any location along the transitory position of the tract from the thyroid gland to the foramen cecum. Spontaneous rupture of the cyst may result in a sinus or fistula.

(Center)   The clear area at the right is a portion of the cyst cavity, which is lined by pseudostratified ciliated columnar epithelium. The circular areas in the connective tissue that are bordered by cuboid cells and filled with a pink-staining, homogeneous, amorphous material are thyroid follicles. Aberrant thyroid tissue, as seen here, is found frequently in the wall of thyroglossal duct cysts, sinuses, and fistulae.

LINGUAL THYROID

(Bottom)   This is a section of a mass that was removed from the undersurface of the tongue because it interfered with deglutition. In the lower portion of the photomicrograph are numerous thyroid follicles. This anomaly is formed from the anterior (lingual) portion of the thyroglossal duct which can form thyroid tissue. Thyroid tissue may have failed to form in its normal location, leaving this tissue as the only functioning thyroid gland. An ^{131}I scan may be used to outline the ectopic gland and to determine whether a normal gland is present. Thyroid neoplasms have been identified in these lingual lesions.

ORAL TORI

A hyperostosis occurring in the midline of the hard palate is termed *torus palatinus,* while one located on the lingual aspect of the mandible in the canine-premolar region is designated *torus mandibularis.* Other localized, nonneoplastic, external bony overgrowths are frequently associated with the maxillary buccal plate, but these hyperostoses usually are not classified as tori.

(Top) A torus palatinus is present at the midline with maxillary hyperostoses on either side. They consist of hard laminated bone with deeper portions of spongy bone. The overlying mucosa usually is very thin, blanched, and easily traumatized. Torus palatinus, of varying sizes, occurs in about 20% of the population, more frequently in adults than in children. It is more common in Asians than in Caucasians or blacks and appears to be genetically determined. Tori and hyperostoses are radiopaque. There is no need to remove the bony prominences unless they interfere with speech or the fitting of dentures or become ulcerated from trauma. Torus palatinus should be differentiated from benign pleomorphic adenomas of the palate, which are firm but not bony hard and which rarely are located directly in the midline.

(Center) Bilateral mandibular tori in the canine and first premolar regions. Mandibular tori may be a source of annoyance if they are of such a configuration that food debris collects beneath them. It is usually necessary to remove them before constructing a denture. They occur less frequently than palatal tori, being found in 8% of the general population, except for some Eskimo groups. Although they are usually bilateral, mandibular tori may be unilateral. They may be unilobular or multilobular, and are radiopaque.

(Bottom) A histologic section from a mandibular torus that is composed entirely of compact bone. The deeper portions of larger tori may contain spongy bone. Histologically, tori and hyperostoses are identical.

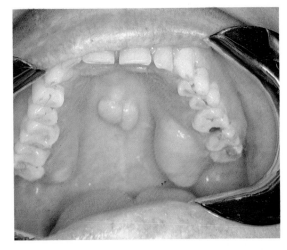

Palatal Torus

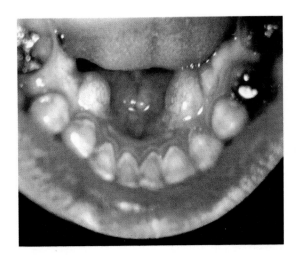

Mandibular Tori

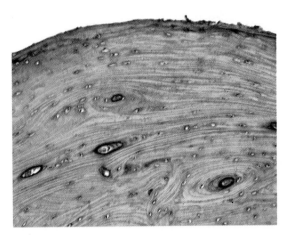

Torus   ×100

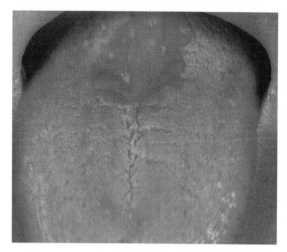

Median Rhomboid Glossitis

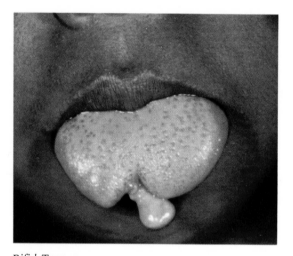

Bifid Tongue

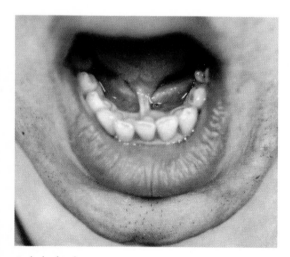

Ankyloglossia

MEDIAN RHOMBOID GLOSSITIS

Median rhomboid glossitis (central papillary atrophy) has been considered a developmental disturbance of the tongue. As shown on pages 12 and 13 the anterior part of the tongue develops from the 1st branchial arch by two lateral prominences and one median prominence (the tuberculum impar). The lateral prominences unite in the midline and overgrow the tuberculum impar. Median rhomboid glossitis has been thought to result from failure of the lateral prominences to overgrow the tuberculum impar. Failure to identify median rhomboid glossitis in infants and the constant presence of *Candida albicans* in the lesions has led to the suggestion that this is an inflammatory lesion rather than a developmental defect. The possibility that the region of the persistent tuberculum impar affords a surface more amenable to colonization of *Candida* should be considered. It is important to note that this benign lesion does not require surgery.

(Top) In this example a smooth, ill-defined, red area appears anterior to the foramen cecum. The lesion is rare (less than 0.4%) and usually is not observed until adult life. It should not be confused with carcinoma, which is even more rare in this location.

BIFID TONGUE

(Center) A midline cleft divides the tip of the tongue into two parts. The tag of tissue seen in the bifurcation consists of muscle. This fairly rare anomaly is the result of the failure of the two lateral halves of the anterior two-thirds of the tongue to fuse completely in the midline and is one of the features of orofacialdigital syndrome.

ANKYLOGLOSSIA

(Bottom) An abnormally broad, short lingual frenum is attached near the tip of this tongue. Tongue-tie of this degree markedly limits the movement of the tongue and may interfere greatly with proper enunciation. This anomaly can be corrected by surgery. However, some individuals overcome their speech problems and learn to enunciate clearly without surgery.

HYPERMOBILE TONGUE

Some individuals have extreme tongue mobility. Such mobility may be congenital or have developed through repeated exercising.

(Top) *(Left)* Protrusion of hypermobile tongue. *(Right)* Tongue positioned behind soft palate in the same patient

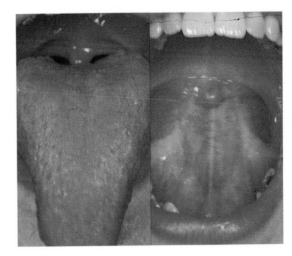

Hypermobile Tongue

MACROGLOSSIA

Macroglossia (large tongue) may be congenital or acquired. Congenital macroglossia may be idiopathic or the result of angiomas and neurofibromas. Acquired macroglossia may be associated with cretinism, myxedema, Down's syndrome, acromegaly, amyloidosis, true muscular hypertrophy, or edema from steroid therapy. Persons who have been edentulous for many years may develop large tongues because of muscular hypertrophy due to the marked use of the tongue to aid in mastication of food. If the patient is able to wear dentures, the tongue muscle may return to normal size.

(Center) Congenital macroglossia due to hemangioma. A 20-month-old girl is unable to retract her tongue into her mouth. The dark crusted tip is exposed continuously. A large tongue was noted at a few days of age, gradually increasing in size with continuously greater exposure. Less frequently, similar changes are produced by lymphangioma. Congenital neurofibroma can produce macroglossia, but in this case the tongue is usually firmer than when enlargement is on a vascular basis, and there is no alteration in color. When hemangioma is the cause, the tongue is bluish; with lymphangioma it is pink or brownish.

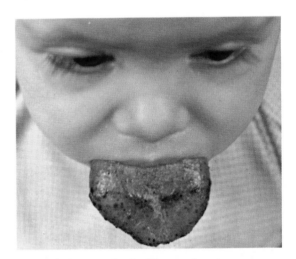

Congenital Macroglossia (Hemangioma)

(Bottom) This tongue with a serrated border from pressure of contacting the teeth displays a typical form of enlargement. (Fissuring with a deep midline pattern is also notable in this instance.) It may be the result of fluid retention in association with generalized disease or may be due to muscular hypertrophy in patients who habitually press the tongue against the teeth. Similar lateral serrations may occur in persons with acromegaly (see p. 137). Recognition of such tongue habits is important in patients with periodontal disease and in patients who are candidates for dentures.

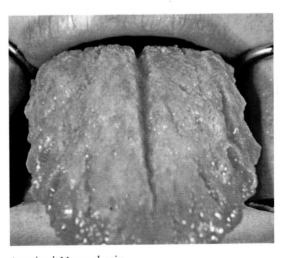

Acquired Macroglossia

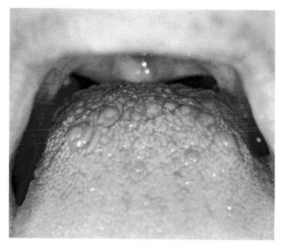

Large Circumvallate Papillae

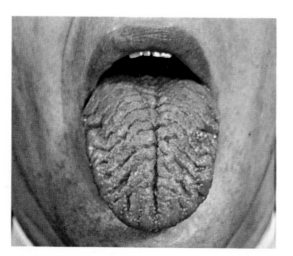

Inflamed Foliate Papillae

ENLARGED LINGUAL PAPILLAE

Large Vallate Papillae

(Top) Overdeveloped vallate papillae (compare normal, p. 5) are plainly visible as large nodules on the dorsum of the tongue. Vallate papillae vary greatly in size, but because they are so far to the posterior, they are not readily visualized unless the tongue is pulled forward.

Foliate Papillae

(Center) The foliate papillae (see p. 5), generally vestigial in humans, may sometimes be seen as vertical folds of mucosa posteriorly on the lateral borders of the tongue. They contain varying amounts of lymphoid tissue. The most posterior ones, which generally are the largest, are identified as *lingual tonsils* (see also p. 20). Lymphoid hyperplasia associated with upper respiratory infections may cause these papillae to become enlarged, red, and tender, as shown here. The lingual changes, which may create a burning sensation, frequently remain after pharyngeal symptoms subside. Any persistent unilateral lesion should be biopsied to establish the diagnosis. Extranodal tonsilar tissue also may be found in the soft palate and the floor of the mouth.

FISSURED TONGUE

(Bottom) This abnormality is found in varying degrees in approximately 5% of the population and is designated as folded, grooved, or scrotal tongue. It is rarely congenital but may appear in childhood or early adult life. Fissured tongue is present in 50% of patients with Melkersson-Rosenthal syndrome, along with intermittent facial nerve palsy and orofacial edema. Prevalence progressively increases in each decade of adult life. This change is of little significance except when the fissures become irritated from retention of debris. The pattern of fissuring varies from symmetrical configurations to irregular haphazard distribution. This illustration demonstrates a tongue with closely adapted deep folds of symmetrical pattern. Visualization is accomplished by having the tongue fully extended and stretched.

Fissured Tongue

(Top)   This picture illustrates an irregular fissured pattern with deep branching grooves. The fungiform papillae are prominent at the borders of the fissures where filiform papillae are absent. The enlarged fungiform papillae are subject to irritation and may become tender. The smooth lighter area at the anterior margin is a healing lesion of benign migratory glossitis (see p. 115). Fissuring of the tongue sometimes is associated with vitamin B complex deficiency.

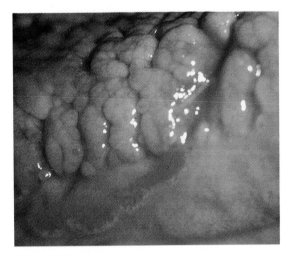

Fissured Tongue

FORDYCE SPOTS (GRANULES)

(Center)   The numerous small, light-yellow macular areas in the buccal mucosa and the upper lip are Fordyce spots. They are sebaceous glands that are in close relation to the covering epithelium. These spots, which are without clinical significance, are found in 82% of the general population. They are seen less frequently in children because, although the sebaceous glands may be present in these locations, they are small and undeveloped; at puberty they become activated and are more prominent and easily observed. Fordyce spots (granules) are usually few in number and discrete, but when they are confluent and involve the whole buccal mucosa, they give it the appearance of chamois skin with a nodular surface. They are found most commonly in the buccal mucosa, the retromolar region, and the lip, but they sometimes occur in the gingiva and the palate. Close inspection of the involved areas will occasionally reveal duct openings from which a greasy substance, sebum, may exude.

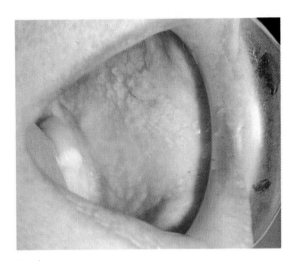

Fordyce Spots

(Bottom)   Section from the buccal mucosa of an individual having clinical evidence of Fordyce spots. At the top of the section is stratified squamous epithelium. Below it in the submucosa are sebaceous gland lobules. Their secretion may help to lubricate the oral mucosa. Sebaceous glands are normally located in the dermis of skin (see p. 2).

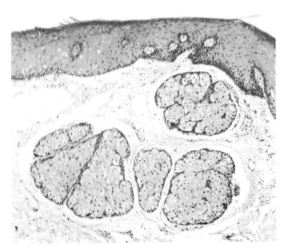

Sebaceous Glands in the Oral Mucosa   ×80

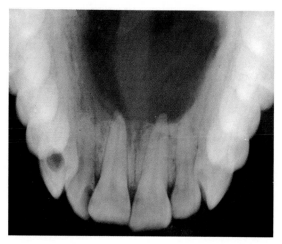

Median Palatine Cyst

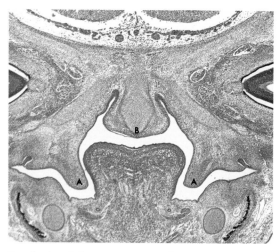

*Developing Palate, Human Embryo
(8 Weeks)   × 30*

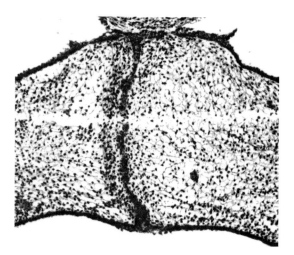

*United Palatine Processes, Human Embryo
(10 Weeks)   × 100*

MEDIAN PALATINE CYST

A median palatine cyst is a fissural cyst originating from epithelium persistent in the embryologic junction of the lateral palatine processes. Its location is in the midline of the palate posterior to the premaxilla.

(Top)   Median palatine cyst revealed in the radiograph as a large, circular radiolucent area in the center of the hard palate. All maxillary teeth in this case tested vital. This cyst bulged into the oral cavity, but many examples of the entity are not evident clinically and are not discovered until routine radiographs are taken. A median palatine, globulomaxillary, or nasopalatine duct cyst, evidenced by radiolucency in a periapical film, may be misinterpreted as a periapical lesion unless further diagnostic procedures, such as pulp testing, are conducted.

(Center)   A frontal section through the head of an 8-week-old human embryo showing that the oral and nasal cavities communicate. The tongue is seen at the bottom of the picture between the lateral palatine processes (*A*), which have not yet united with each other, or with the nasal septum (*B*).

(Bottom)   Section from a 10-week-old embryo cut in the same plane as the one in the center picture, showing a later stage of development. The lateral palatine processes have now joined with each other and with the nasal septum above. The vertical line of union in the center of the photomicrograph consists of a double row of dark-staining epithelial cells. On each side of this line is lacelike mesenchymal tissue that should perforate and obliterate the epithelium, making the union complete. If any of the epithelial cells remain in the midline, they may give rise to a median palatine cyst. The upper portion of this epithelium has the potential to differentiate into pseudostratified ciliated columnar epithelium, the lower portion into the stratified squamous variety. Therefore, a cyst developing in this region may be lined by either or both types, depending on which epithelial cells are entrapped.

GLOBULOMAXILLARY CYST

The globulomaxillary cyst has been considered to result from epithelium persisting at the place of union of the globular portion of the median nasal process with the maxillary process. The cyst appears between the roots of the lateral incisor and those of the canine. The developmental origin has been questioned, and an origin from odontogenic epithelium proposed. The exact origin is somewhat academic since treatment in either case is surgical removal.

(Top) A pear-shaped radiolucency is seen in an occlusal radiograph between the roots of the lateral incisor and of the canine. Normal pulp vitality of the teeth and divergence of their roots are diagnostic points in differentiating this cyst from an apical periodontal cyst but not from a lateral developmental cyst (see p. 33). If the pulps are not involved, the cyst should be enucleated without sacrificing adjacent teeth.

(Center) Photomicrograph of a portion of a cyst removed from the globulomaxillary area. The cyst cavity is lined by a thin layer of stratified squamous epithelium. Most cysts of this region are not lined by pseudostratified columnar epithelium, which has led to questioning of the developmental origin theory.

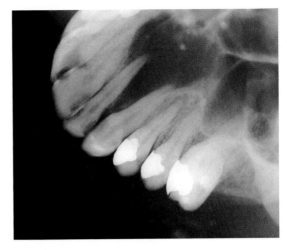

Globulomaxillary Radiolucency

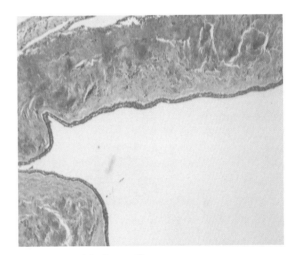

Cyst from Globulomaxillary Area × 100

NASOLABIAL CYST

(Bottom) A nasolabial cyst is formed from epithelial remnants at the junction of the medial nasal, the lateral nasal, and the maxillary processes. It is found in the soft tissue above the canine-lateral incisor region, usually on the surface of the maxilla. This cyst may cause a bulge in the floor of the nose or on the face. It may be misdiagnosed as an extension of a dentoalveolar abscess or an abscess formed in an infected hair follicle within the naris. The diagnosis of nasolabial cyst can be confirmed by aspirating the fluid, replacing it with radiopaque media, and radiographing.

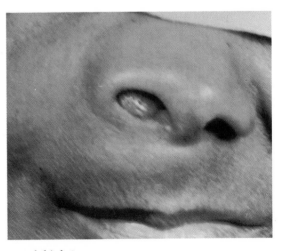

Nasolabial Cyst

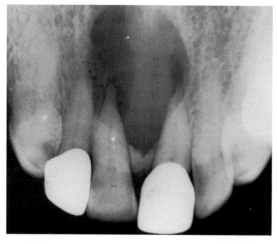

Nasopalatine Duct Cyst

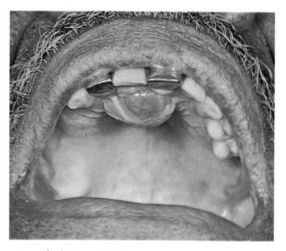

Nasopalatine Duct Cyst

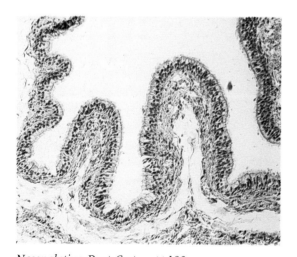

Nasopalatine Duct Cyst   × 100

NASOPALATINE DUCT CYST

After the palatine processes unite, as shown on page 28, and meet with the premaxilla anteriorly, there is still communication between the oral and nasal cavities by two epithelium-lined tubes, the nasopalatine ducts. These structures are located immediately to each side of the midline above the area that later will be the palatine papilla. In lower animals they are primordia of a pair of accessory olfactory organs, but in humans they serve no useful purpose and ordinarily obliterate. If any portion of these ducts persists, the remaining epithelium may be the source of a nasopalatine duct (incisive canal) cyst.

(Top)   The cyst is represented by the circular radiolucent area in the incisive canal region. It is situated distal to the roots of the central incisors. The pulps of anterior teeth in this patient tested vital. A nasopalatine duct cyst may be located to one side of the midline if its origin is epithelial debris from only one of the ducts.

(Center)   The marked swelling, as seen in the region of the palatine papilla, is caused by the nasopalatine duct cyst shown above, which was both intra- and extraosseous. Extraosseous cysts are termed *cysts of the palatine papilla.*

(Bottom)   The nasopalatine duct cyst may be lined by pseudostratified ciliated columnar epithelium, stratified squamous epithelium, or a modification of both. Mucous glands, hyaline cartilage, large vessels, and nerves may be found in the cyst wall. Inflammatory cells are uncommon. In this photomicrograph of a nasopalatine duct cyst the cyst cavity is lined by pseudostratified columnar epithelium.

DENTIGEROUS CYST

The dentigerous cyst develops about the crown of an unerupted tooth after amelogenesis is completed. It may involve the entire crown (central type) or only a portion of it (lateral type). The dentigerous cyst usually develops outside the ameloblastic layer. It may arise between the ameloblastic layer and either the stratum intermedium or the outer enamel epithelium or from cells proliferating from the odontogenic epithelium or from remnants of the dental lamina. In such instances it is lined entirely by epithelium. It is possible that a dentigerous cyst may result from fluid accumulating between the ameloblasts and the enamel, in which case the odontogenic epithelium lines the outer portions of the cyst with enamel centrally. The term *dentigerous cyst* is sometimes applied to cysts which develop about odontomas.

Both dentigerous and primordial cysts (see p. 32) are sometimes classified as follicular cysts. The term *eruption cyst* is used for a dentigerous cyst that is in a superficial position over the crown of a tooth and manifested clinically by a bulging of the overlying mucosa. It may contain some blood and be mistaken, on cursory examination, for a hemangioma or hematoma.

(Top) Central dentigerous cyst enveloping the crown of a mandibular 3rd molar. Note that the involved 3rd molar is depressed inferiorly. All lesions appearing radiographically as dentigerous cysts should be examined histologically to rule out ameloblastoma (see p. 152).

(Center) Radiograph of a lateral dentigerous cyst, involving only the distal portion of the crown. This should not be confused with a lateral periodontal cyst, which does not involve the crown (see p. 33).

(Bottom) Third molar tooth with dentigerous cyst enveloping the crown. The space between the tooth crown and cyst wall contained fluid. Note that the crown is fully developed. All dentigerous cysts should be submitted for pathologic examination to rule out the possibility of ameloblastoma developing from the lining epithelium.

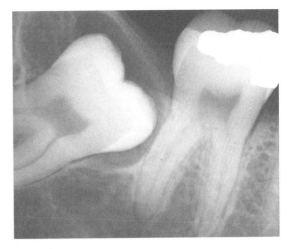

Central Dentigerous Cyst

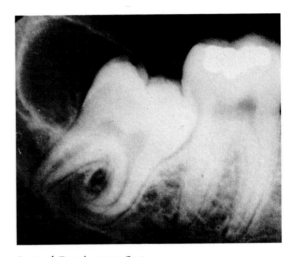

Lateral Dentigerous Cyst

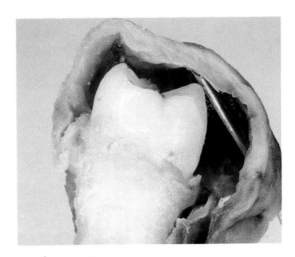

Dentigerous Cyst

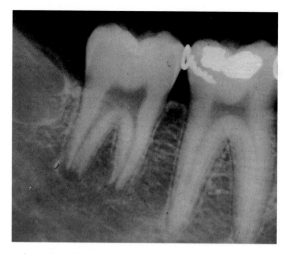

Primordial Cyst

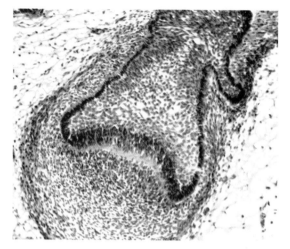

Developing Tooth × 150

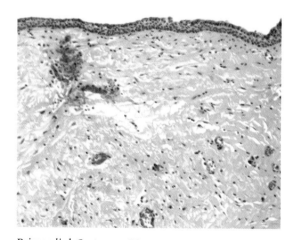

Primordial Cyst × 90

PRIMORDIAL CYST

The primordial cyst develops because of cystic degeneration of the bud, cap, or early bell stage of an enamel organ. Because this metamorphosis occurs before the enamel organ has initiated induction of hard dental tissues, this cyst always arises in place of, rather than in relationship with, a tooth. It is the least common of odontogenic cysts, occurring most often in the mandibular 3rd molar region. Examination and history demonstrate its presence in place of one of the 3rd molars. This cyst formerly was classified as a follicular cyst because of its origin within the dental follicle.

(Top) Radiograph of the 3rd molar region of a 13-year-old boy shows a radiolucent area in place of a calcifying 3rd molar. The other 3rd molars were present. Histologic examination of the surgical specimen revealed findings compatible with clinical diagnosis of primordial cyst.

(Center) At this stage of tooth development, or even earlier (see p. 14), the stellate reticulum may degenerate as a result of trauma, infection, or some other factor. As the cells of the stellate reticulum liquefy, the remaining inner and outer enamel epithelia form a sac. This fluid-filled sac, with its connective tissue capsule, is the primordial cyst. Tooth development cannot proceed, but the cyst may enlarge slowly.

(Bottom) The cyst cavity (clear area at top) is lined for the most part with compressed stratified squamous epithelium. The lining at the right, however, somewhat resembles odontogenic epithelium. In this case the connective tissue cyst wall is conspicuously devoid of any inflammatory elements. Ordinarily, a primordial cyst cannot be distinguished histologically from other types of cysts seen in the jaw. However, a number of these have been reported as keratocysts (see p. 34). To determine that a cyst is of the primordial variety, it is necessary that the histologic findings be supplemented by the clinical history and the radiologic examination.

DEVELOPMENTAL LATERAL PERIODONTAL CYST

(Top) This is a relatively rare form of odontogenic cyst that occurs in the periodontal ligament alongside a vital tooth. It appears radiographically similar to the inflammatory periodontal cyst (see pp. 68, 69) but is not associated with a lateral branch of the pulp canal or with inflammation of periodontal origin. If it occurs between the lateral incisor and canine, it may be considered a globulomaxillary cyst (p. 29). Some cysts in this location may be primordial cysts of supernumerary tooth buds; others may arise from epithelial rests of Malassez.

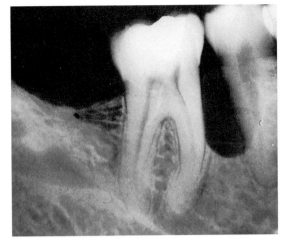

Lateral Periodontal Cyst

(Center) Photomicrograph of a section of tooth with an attached lateral periodontal cyst. In the lower left corner a portion of the pulp canal can be seen. To the right of this area there is dentin, then a thin line of cementum, and finally a mass of fibrous connective tissue containing inflammatory cells. In this connective tissue is a cyst cavity lined by dark-blue-staining stratified squamous epithelium. There was no evidence of pulpal inflammation.

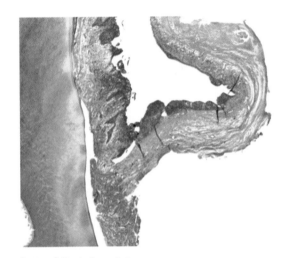

Lateral Periodontal Cyst   × 100

CALCIFYING ODONTOGENIC CYST

(Bottom) Photomicrograph of calcifying (and keratinizing) odontogenic cyst. These cysts are lined by squamous epithelium that forms masses of keratin in which large "ghost" epithelial cells are trapped. The degenerated ghost cells undergo calcification. Odontogenic type epithelium is in evidence. The cyst may be either intra- or extraosseous. Radiographically the lesions are radiolucent with radiopaque flecks that vary with the degree of intracystic calcification. It is believed that the lesion, although cystic, is related to the epithelial odontogenic tumors. There is some tendency to recurrence after surgical treatment.

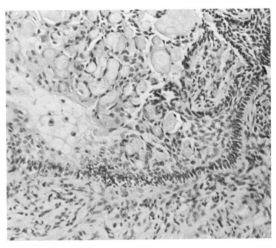

Calcifying Odontogenic Cyst   × 100

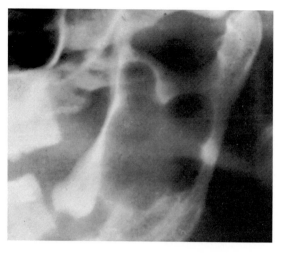

Odontogenic Keratocyst (Dentigerous Cyst Type)

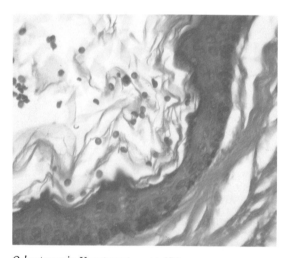

Odontogenic Keratocyst × 450

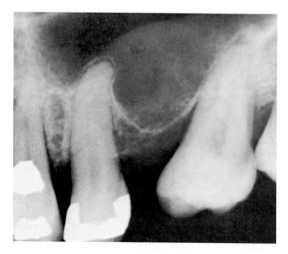

Pseudocyst of Maxillary Sinus

ODONTOGENIC KERATOCYST

The term *odontogenic keratocyst* refers to those cysts of odontogenic origin in which the lining stratified squamous epithelium uniformly produces keratin. The clinical behavior of these cysts is considerably different from the other types of odontogenic cysts in that they tend to be more aggressive and tend to recur following removal. Keratinized linings may occur in primordial cysts, dentigerous cysts, lateral periodontal cysts, and occasionally in apical periodontal cysts. In addition, multiple keratocysts may form one of the components of nevoid basal cell carcinoma syndrome.

(Top) Radiograph of large dentigerous cyst involving body of mandible and extending just inferior to the coronoid notch. Histologic examination revealed this to be an odontogenic keratocyst of dentigerous cyst type.

(Center) Photomicrograph of odontogenic keratocyst showing keratin production by the lining epithelium. The lining also may invaginate (producing "daughter cysts") and, when incompletely curetted, produce recurrences.

MUCOCELES AND PSEUDOCYSTS OF MAXILLARY SINUS

(Bottom)Radiograph of pseudocyst. Note the characteristic dome-shaped lesion. Cysts and cystlike processes arising from sinus mucosa include (1) *Pseudocysts.* These represent focal accumulations of inflammatory exudate that lift the antral mucosa away from underlying bone. (2) Retention cysts of the seromucinous glands. These are seldom large enough to be evident radiographically. (3) Mucoceles, which represent herniations of the antral lining through the sinus wall. These are destructive lesions. Some are caused by obstruction of the ostium; others are secondary to to surgery, usually the Caldwell-Luc procedure.

GEMINATION AND FUSION

Geminated teeth are formed by the partial "twinning" of a single tooth germ. The two resulting components may be approximately equal in size, or one may be rudimentary in size and form. While the term *gemination* may be applied properly to the formation of twin teeth that are separate entities, usually it is reserved for those instances of maldevelopment in which only partial cleavage of the tooth germ has occurred. Geminated teeth usually have a single root and a common pulp canal. Clinically, the normal number of teeth can be accounted for in the dentition, counting the bifid tooth as one.

(Top) Gemination in which the double tooth developed from the formative organ of the maxillary right lateral incisor. The maxillary dentition consists of a normal number of teeth, the presence of an unerupted canine being revealed by radiologic examination. Clinical evidence of this fact is also apparent from the bulge above the edentulous area.

(Center) Fused teeth result from the union of two adjacent tooth germs. The two teeth may be united for their entire length or joined only by their crowns or their roots. The fusion must involve the dentin, for when two teeth are connected only by cementum, the condition is termed concrescence (see p. 39).

(Bottom) Radiograph of the fused incisors shown in the center photograph. The dentin of the two teeth is continuous and there appears to be a division of the coronal pulp chambers. Fusion of primary teeth is more common than fusion of permanent teeth, although both are rare.

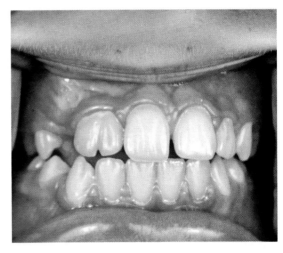

Gemination

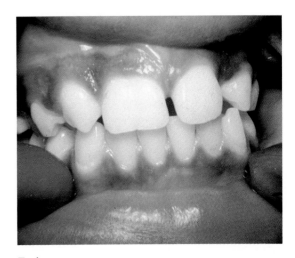

Fusion

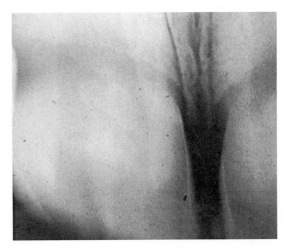

Fusion

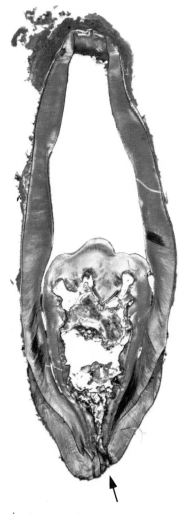

Dens Invaginatus ×6

DENS INVAGINATUS

(DENS IN DENTE)

This anomaly appears radiographically as a "tooth within a tooth." Actually it is formed by the retarded growth of a portion of a single tooth germ or by the proliferation of a segment of the odontogenic epithelium into the dental papilla. Also known as dens in dente or gestant anomaly, it usually involves a maxillary lateral incisor. A communication exists between the oral cavity and the enamel-lined inner cavity which can be considered as an extremely deep pit. Debris and bacteria may accumulate in this inner cavity, and caries usually develops unnoticed. For this reason pulpitis and periapical inflammation are commonly associated with dens invaginatus. This anomaly may be discovered in routine radiographic examinations or because pain occurs in an apparently intact tooth.

(Top) A ground section of a dens invaginatus in a maxillary lateral incisor photographed in polarized light. Near the tip of the cusp, in the lower part of the picture, a small opening into the inner cavity may be seen *(arrow)*. At midcrown the structures may be observed from the surface to the center on either side in the following order: enamel, dentin, thin slitlike space occupied by pulp, dentin, enamel, central cavity space. A similar anomaly occurring in the roots may present a central cavity lined by cementum rather than enamel.

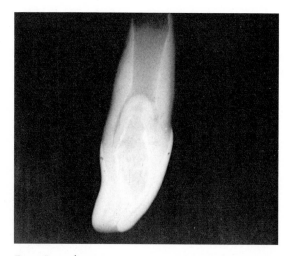

Dens Invaginatus

(Bottom) Radiograph of maxillary second incisor with dens invaginitus. The pulp chamber divides into two narrow horns on either side of the invagination. At the incisal edge a communication with the pear-shaped enamel lined cavity can be identified. Through this type of opening cariogenic bacteria and carbohydrates may enter the invaginated cavity and cause dental caries and pulpal involvement.

MICRODONTIA

(Top) Example of a very small tooth (microdontia, dwarfism). Such variations in size may occur in single teeth, a few teeth, or all teeth of a given dentition. When all teeth are large or small, but proportionate to the general constitution, they may be considered as normal. Gigantism of individual teeth is most frequent in the incisor or canine region, while 3rd molars and maxillary lateral incisors are the teeth most frequently dwarfed. The maxillary lateral incisors may be peg-shaped. Both large and small teeth tend to occur in pairs and often follow a genetic pattern although other factors may be active (see p. 104, *center*).

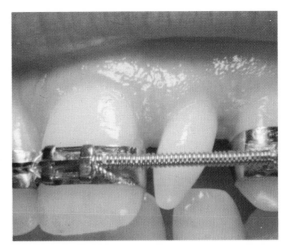

Microdontia

SUPERNUMERARY TEETH

(Center) A supernumerary tooth with the crown form of a premolar has displaced the maxillary right central incisor and prevented the eruption of the right lateral. Supernumerary teeth, in addition to interfering with normal eruption, may be situated between the roots of adjacent teeth, causing a diastema; they may erupt into the buccal or lingual embrasures and also may occur outside of the normal line of the dental arch. These extra teeth are observed most frequently in the maxillary incisor and the 3rd molar regions. They are produced as a result of accessory tooth buds differentiating from the dental lamina. Even when erupted, supernumerary teeth are often unobserved or overlooked.

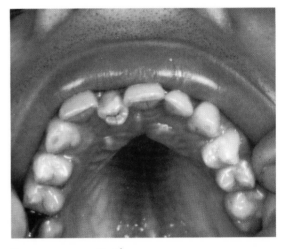

Supernumerary Tooth

(Bottom) A radiograph showing a median diastema caused by an unerupted supernumerary tooth. The term *mesiodens* is sometimes applied to a tooth in this location because it is mesial to the two central incisors. Teeth that occur distally to 3rd molars are designated as *distomolars,* while those appearing laterally may be called *paramolars.* Among the explanations proposed for the appearance of supernumerary teeth in the incisor and the premolar regions is reversion to the typical mammalian formula of six incisors and eight premolars in either jaw.

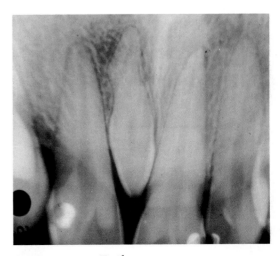

Supernumerary Tooth

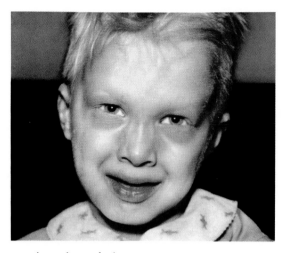

Ectodermal Dysplasia

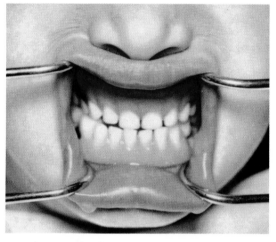

Complete Anodontia

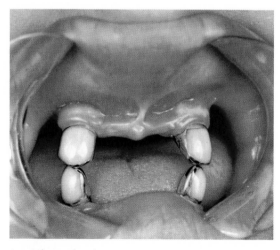

Partial Anodontia

ECTODERMAL DYSPLASIA

This genetic disease of faulty ectodermal development is inherited most frequently as an X-linked recessive trait. It is characterized by a few or many of the following abnormalities: lack of sweat and sebaceous glands; smooth, atrophic skin; total or partial anodontia; defective hair, nail, and iris formation; atrophic rhinitis; deficiency of lacrimal, pharyngeal, conjunctival, and salivary glands; prominent forehead; saddle-type nose; thick lips, and dysphonia. In the anhidrotic and hypohydrotic types, the inability to perspire greatly interferes with the well-being of the individual because the heat-regulating mechanism cannot keep the body at the proper temperature.

(Top) A 5-year-old boy exhibiting manifestations of ectodermal dysplasia. He has very fine, sparse, silken hair and scant eyebrows and eyelashes; frontal eminences are quite prominent, and the nose is depressed at the root. The skin is smooth and glossy, and the lips are thick. Abnormality was first suspected at 8 mo, when teeth had not yet appeared. Shortly thereafter, with the advent of warm weather, the child felt hot, showed signs of distress, and had an unusual thirst. When he was placed in an air-conditioned room, these symptoms abated.

(Center) Intraoral view of the above patient wearing complete artificial dentures, the lower one being slightly dislodged by the cheek retractor. Radiographs did not reveal tooth buds of either the primary or the permanent dentition. At the corners of the nose the dryness and thinness of the skin are well demonstrated. This patient has neither rhinitis nor a deficiency in salivary flow but does have a constant rough quality of voice.

(Bottom) Another case of ectodermal dysplasia, characterized by hypotrichosis, anhidrosis, photophobia, and partial anodontia. Mild partial anodontia (congenital absence of one or two pair of teeth) is a relatively common defect in the general population and is not usually associated with ectodermal dysplasia. When all or most of the teeth are missing, however, the syndrome should be suspected.

CONCRESCENCE

The term *concrescence* denotes the *cemental* union of two fully formed teeth that originally were separate entities. Two factors are essential for this condition: (1) excessive deposition of cementum and (2) close approximation of the roots of adjacent teeth. The process is similar to that which occurs when a fractured root is repaired (see p. 56). Concrescence differs from fusion in that the union in the latter results in coalescence of respective dentins (see p. 35). Concrescence is observed most frequently in the maxillary molar region.

(Top)   An example of concrescence. The root of a 2nd molar is joined by cementum to the root of a 3rd molar that was completely unerupted.

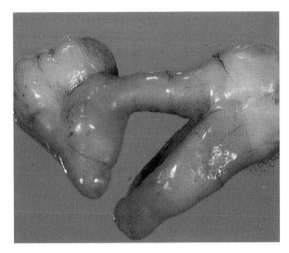

Concrescence

HYPERCEMENTOSIS

The formation of excessive cementum on the root may be due to trauma, local or general (see p. 129) metabolic dysfunction, periapical inflammation, as compensation for occlusal movement, or a defect in development. The excessive cementum is formed in layers. If cells are entrapped in the matrix, it is termed *cellular cementum.*

(Center)   Radiograph showing two premolars with hypercementosis. The periodontal ligament space is clearly present around both tooth roots.

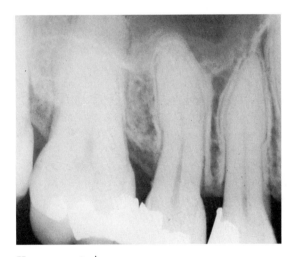

Hypercementosis

(Bottom)   Photomicrograph of a tooth with hypercementosis involving the apical third of the root. The periodontal ligament is evident between the cementum and the surrounding alveolar bone. Hypercementosis may be limited to one or a few teeth or may be generalized.

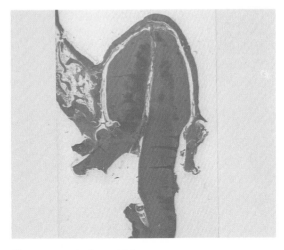

Hypercementosis   × 6

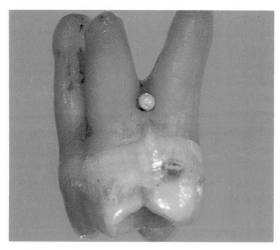

Enamel Pearl

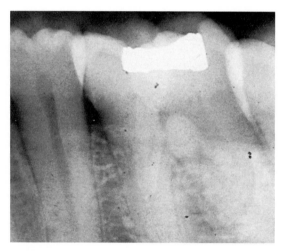

Enamel Pearl

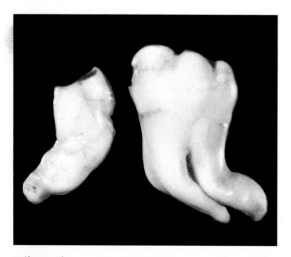

Dilaceration

ENAMEL PEARLS

Enamel pearls (nodulous anomalies, enamel drops, enamelomas) are small masses of enamel found apically to the amelocemental junction. They occur most frequently at the bifurcation of molar roots and may appear in radiographs as round radiopacities. Their presence is of clinical significance only when gingival recession or periodontal disease involves the bifurcation or root surface supporting the enamel pearl. These anomalies probably form when a portion of Hertwig's sheath remains in contact with the dentin and is stimulated to differentiate into functional ameloblasts.

(Top) This molar (maxillary) has a large pearl in the bifurcation area.

(Center) Radiograph of a mandibular molar with an enamel pearl at its bifurcation. These are not rare but they are frequently overlooked or not recorded, probably because they are innocuous.

DILACERATION

Dilaceration, technically, refers to distortion of the root or crown caused by a tearing during tooth development with a resultant crease at the point of distortion and a very sharp bend. Through usage the term is now used for any severe angulation with distortion of the roots such as that seen in mandibular 3rd molars distorted by lack of space for development. The roots of all posterior teeth tend to have a distal inclination, but the term dilaceration should be used only for sharp distortions.

(Bottom) A dilacerated tooth which may have resulted from an injury to the tooth germ (*left*), and one which may have occurred because of insufficient space in which to develop (*right*).

ENAMEL DYSPLASIA

Enamel dysplasia is a broad term encompassing two types of abnormal enamel development: enamel hypoplasia and enamel hypocalcification. Enamel hypoplasia may be produced by any disturbance severe enough to interfere with ameloblastic function during formation of enamel matrix (apposition of enamel). Enamel hypocalcification may be caused by any factor that inhibits enamel maturation (the calcification of enamel). Local, systemic, or hereditary disturbances may be etiologic factors in either type. Local factors such as periapical inflammation or trauma to a deciduous tooth may cause either hypoplasia or hypocalcification of the permanent successor. Nutritional deficiencies (particularly of vitamins A and D), endocrine dysfunction, and generalized infection during odontogenesis are among the systemic causes. An excessive amount of fluorides in the drinking water during odontogenesis is the most common cause of hypocalcification. The term *amelogenesis imperfecta* is applied to hereditary types of enamel dysplasia.

(Top) Severe hypoplasia with pits and grooves at different levels on different teeth. The defects occur in the enamel that was being formed at the time of the disturbance. An exanthematous fever is often considered as the specific systemic factor responsible for this form of hypoplasia, but investigation will often reveal that the time of interruption of amelogenesis does not correspond to the time period of the disease.

(Center) Enamel hypoplasia caused by periapical inflammation of a primary tooth extending into permanent tooth bud at 6 years of age. These sometimes are termed *Turner's teeth*.

(Bottom) Almost total aplasia of enamel in the lower incisors and canines. There is a small amount of enamel near the gingiva on the lower right canine and a sharp ridge demarcating its border. These teeth do not show attrition because of the open bite. The maxillary anterior teeth, now replaced by a partial denture, were affected similarly.

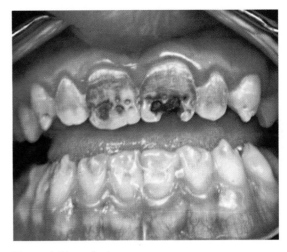

Enamel Hypoplasia

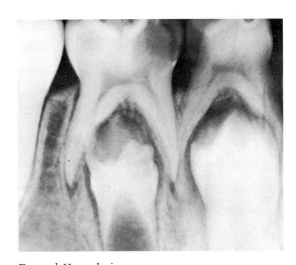

Enamel Hypoplasia

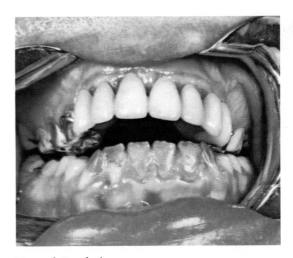

Enamel Dysplasia

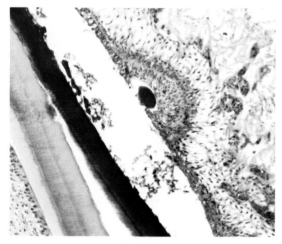

Enamel Hypoplasia   × 100

ENAMEL DYSPLASIA *(continued)*

(Top) Photomicrograph of a developing tooth from a 43-day-old infant born 3 mo prematurely. The diagonal clear space in the center is an artifact separating the enamel organ (right) from the previously formed blue-staining enamel matrix. To the right of the artifact, partially surrounding a globule of abnormal enamel matrix, is a proliferation of poorly differentiated cells. This proliferation of odontogenic epithelium is apparently a reparative procedure—an attempt to replace degenerated ameloblasts. The cells in this zone are probably nonfunctional, and the area would have been represented clinically as a pit or groove.

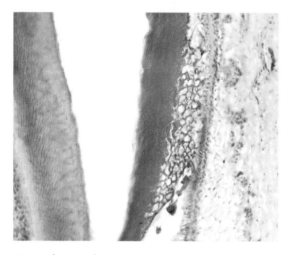

Enamel Hypoplasia   × 100

(Center) In this photomicrograph from the same patient, the V-shaped clear space is an artifact. Proceeding to the right from the artifact is first a reddish band of normal enamel matrix, next a vacuolated area, and then a row of ameloblasts. It is believed that the foamy enamel matrix (vacuolated area), caused by some disturbance to the ameloblasts, would have been reflected in the clinical appearance of the tooth as a hypoplastic defect.

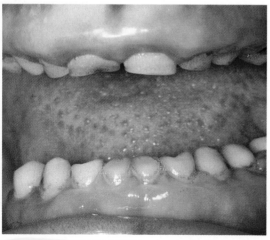
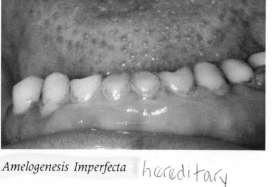

Amelogenesis Imperfecta   hereditary

(Bottom) This example of enamel dysplasia is designated as *amelogenesis imperfecta* since the abnormality was exhibited by several members of the family as a dominant nonsex-linked mendelian trait. Some members of these families may show minor dysplastic effects in other ectodermal structures. This patient exhibits abnormal enamel formation ranging from complete absence of enamel to deposition of incompletely matured enamel matrix. Complete failure of enamel formation is apparent on the maxillary incisors.

(Top) Periapical radiograph of teeth affected by amelogenesis imperfecta. Crown and root formation appear normal, but no enamel is present on the tooth crowns. Teeth so affected do not exhibit an increased susceptibility to dental caries. All teeth in both arches were affected.

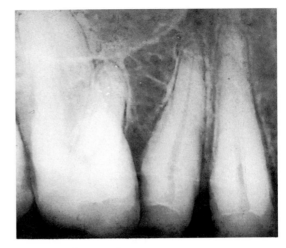

Amelogenesis Imperfecta

(Center) A mild case of mottled enamel (endemic dental fluorosis), which is an acquired form of enamel hypocalcification caused by the consumption of water having an excessive amount of fluorine. To cause mottling, the water must contain more than one part per million of the element and be consumed during the period of tooth development. The fluorine, unless in extremely high concentration, does not injure the ameloblasts sufficiently to interfere with enamel apposition, but the matrix formed by such ameloblasts does not mature completely. When decalcified microscopic sections are made of mature enamel, which is acid-soluble, only a scant amount of matrix may be seen. When teeth with mottled enamel are likewise prepared, a considerable amount of enamel matrix is apparent in the brown areas. Because this hypocalcified enamel is high in organic content, it is relatively acid-resistant and appears microscopically not unlike young enamel matrix of a developing tooth, depicted at the top of p. 6. When teeth of this type originally erupt, there are cloudy, opaque areas, but these porous regions gradually absorb extrinsic material and assume a yellow or brown color.

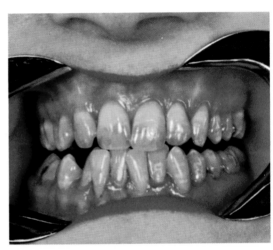

Mottled Enamel Fluorosis

(Bottom) The single chalky-white opaque spot in the left maxillary central incisor is an example of focal hypomaturation (nonendemic mottling) of enamel. The groove above the area of hypocalcification reflects a disturbance in matrix formation. Not all white spots are examples of hypomaturation. Some may be due to altered matrix apposition, which changes the index of refraction. Decalcification in the early phases of dental caries may produce a similar-appearing white spot.

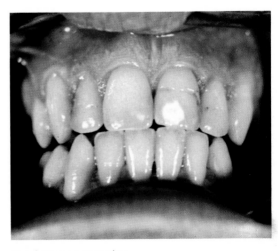

Focal Hypomaturation

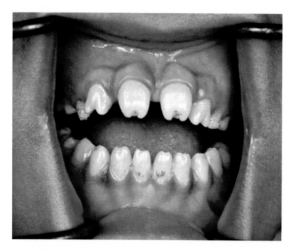

Hutchinson's Incisors

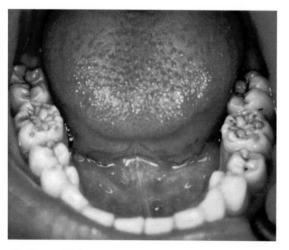

Mulberry Molars

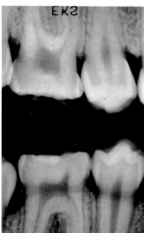

Mulberry Molars　　*Hutchinson's Incisors*

ENAMEL DYSPLASIA *(continued)*

Enamel hypoplasia of both dentitions may result from prenatal syphilis. In the permanent teeth this specific infection also interferes with morpho-differentiation and dentinogenesis. The enamel organ may be directly invaded by *Treponema pallidum*, or may be secondarily affected by inflammatory processes in the surrounding tissues. The spirochete does not enter the fetal circulation until after the 16th week, and its effect on tooth development does not extend beyond early infancy; therefore, only those stages of odontogenesis that occur during this period can be affected. Since morphodifferentiation of the deciduous teeth has already been completed by the 16th wk, their size and shape cannot be altered, but enamel apposition may be disturbed and result in hypoplastic defects that, although caused by syphilis, are not especially pathognomonic of the disease. The permanent teeth (12 anteriors and 4 first molars) are so distinctively affected, when involved, that clinically they can be consistently recognized.

(Top) Typical Hutchinson's incisors in a patient affected by prenatal syphilis. They are notched, screwdriver-shaped teeth with rounded incisal angles. Although faulty matrix formation often accentuates the notch, the abnormal contour is mainly due to alteration in the ameloblastic layer at the time of morphodifferentiation. Hutchinson considered such teeth together with keratitis and nerve deafness as a triad characteristic of congenital syphilis.

(Center) One of the types of 1st molars seen in this disease. Hypoplasia of the enamel, along with the altered shape, gives the occlusal surface a mulberry-like appearance. A variation characterized by a clinched appearance of the crown is known as the bud molar. Attrition of both these types may result in a flat-surfaced tooth with exposed dentin.

(Bottom) Bitewing radiographs showing the characteristic notching and converging lateral borders of the anterior teeth and the marked hypoplasia of the enamel on the occlusal surfaces of the 1st molars. Diagnosis of congenital syphilis should not be based on dental defects alone (see p. 92).

DEFECTS OF DENTIN FORMATION

Dentinogenesis Imperfecta

(HEREDITARY OPALESCENT DENTIN)

This dentinal anomaly is a non-sex-linked genetic disturbance characterized by violet- to amber-colored teeth that have an opalescent iridescence in certain lights, rapid obliteration of the pulp chambers and canals, and severe attrition. It occurs in both the permanent and primary dentition. The enamel tends to chip or shear away from the dentin, and the dentinoenamel junction is smoother than in normal teeth. Histologically and chemically the enamel is normal, but the dentin is very atypical. Dentinal tubules are few in number and of large diameter; they are arranged haphazardly and may appear at right angles to the normal direction. The dentin is poorly calcified with occasional cellular inclusions. It is softer and has a greater water and inorganic content than normal dentin.

(Top)   Dentinogenesis imperfecta in a young patient with attrition of the maxillary incisors that would be excessive for normal teeth at this age. The teeth are opalescent with a violet hue. Almost complete obliteration of the pulp chambers and root canals was demonstrated radiographically.

(Center)   Dentinogenesis imperfecta in a young patient showing severe attrition of the primary teeth. Here the incisor teeth appear purplish-brown and the canines more violet. Probably these variations in color are due to different dentin compositions and, in part, to the angle at which light strikes the enamel surfaces. The excessive wear followed the chipping of enamel from the functional surfaces. The radiographic appearance in this case was typical for dentinogenesis imperfecta.

(Bottom)   Low magnification (*left*) shows normal thin layer of cementum at top, relatively normal outer layer of dentin, and irregularly formed dentin below. The blue lines in the center are due to matrix failure and compression of many dentinal fibers. Under higher power (*right*) the irregular pattern is evident. Tubules of normal size and arrangement are seen at the center. Nodular areas show cross sections of large tubules, irregular tubules, and atubular matrix. As the pulp chambers and root canals are rapidly filled with calcified, but irregular, dentin, they are soon obliterated radiographically. This is important diagnostically.

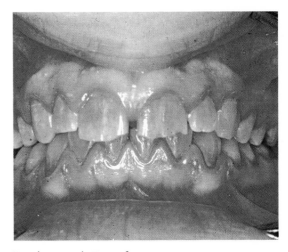

Dentinogenesis Imperfecta

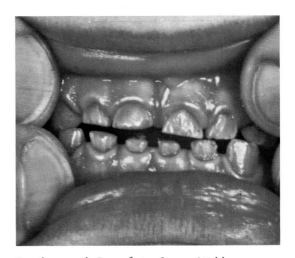

Dentinogenesis Imperfecta, Severe Attrition

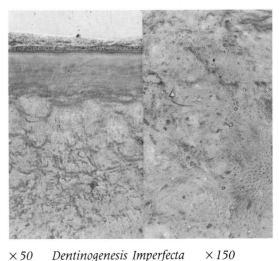

× 50   *Dentinogenesis Imperfecta*   × 150

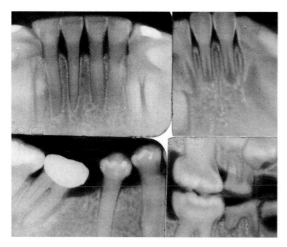

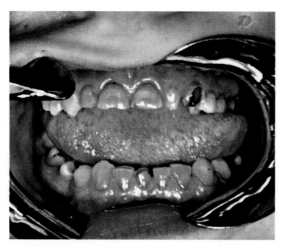

Dentinogenesis Imperfecta

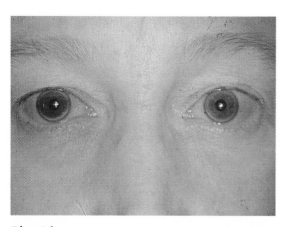

Dentinogenesis Imperfecta in Patient with Osteogenesis Imperfecta

DEFECTS OF DENTIN FORMATION
(continued)

These teeth are usually quite caries-resistant. The sensitivity of the teeth is usually low or negative, but occasionally they give normal responses to pulp tests. Because of their relatively thin roots, they may be prone to root fracture, although they have been successfully treated by jacket and full-veneer crowns.

(Top)   These radiographs are of the same patient at 7 years of age (*right*) and at 17 years (*left*). The upper right shows obliteration of incisal pulp chambers and obliteration of root canals. The lower right illustrates involvement of both dentitions with severe attrition of deciduous molars and obliteration of pulp chambers in deciduous and permanent teeth. The upper left demonstrates complete obliteration of pulp chambers and heavy incisal wear. The lower left shows obliteration of pulp chambers, but a pulp canal may be seen in the distal root of the 2d molar. Because of excessive wear the 1st molar was lost, and the 2d molar required a crown.

(Center)   Osteogenesis imperfecta (brittle bone disease) is a genetically dominant disease manifested by multiple fractures associated with osteoblastic dysfunction or reduction in osteoblasts. It may occur concomitantly with dentinogenesis imperfecta, blue sclerae, or otosclerosis, or any of these may appear alone in a single family or individual. This 14-year-old girl had both dentinogenesis imperfecta and osteogenesis imperfecta. She had over 20 fractures of the legs with marked deformity. The teeth have the characteristic color and show attrition and shearing of the enamel. The pulp chambers and canals were practically obliterated.

(Bottom)   Blue sclerae may occur with osteogenesis imperfecta. The blue color is due to the dark choroid showing through a thin sclera. Patients with osteogenesis imperfecta frequently have concomitant dentinogenesis imperfecta. It is more common, however, for dentinogenesis imperfecta to occur by itself as an isolated genetic condition.

Blue Sclerae

DENTIN DYSPLASIA

Dentin dysplasia is a form of mesenchymal dysplasia now generally considered to be an entity distinct from dentinogenesis imperfecta. It differs from the latter in that the teeth are of normal color; there is no tendency for the enamel to chip off and no rapid attrition; and there is altered, retarded, or deficient root formation with radiolucent areas at the apices of some teeth. It is similar to dentinogenesis imperfecta because of early obliteration of pulp chambers and root canals by atypical dentin.

(Top) Clinical picture of dentin dysplasia. The teeth are of normal color with no attrition. Looseness, malposition, and early loss of teeth may be attributed to retarded root formation and lack of supporting bone.

(Center) Radiographs of patient in top picture are on the right. They show normally shaped crowns, obliteration of pulp chambers, retarded root formation, and apical radiolucencies. The radiographs on the left (from another patient) show sharply defined periapical radiolucencies, absence of pulp chambers and canals, and roots that are better formed but still defective. Sometimes horizontal radiolucencies are seen in the tooth crowns. The apical areas are fibrous but may become inflamed via periodontal pockets, especially on short-rooted teeth, and may develop into abscesses, granulomas, or cysts.

(Bottom) In the decalcified section (without enamel) the only normal dentin is on the periphery. The remainder, which nearly obliterates the pulp chamber, is quite bizarre. Numerous horizontal crescent-shaped clear areas are evident. At higher magnification it is observed that dentin with large tubules curves around nodules of atubular dentin. The apical ends of the nodules are poorly defined, and tubular dentin appears to stream out of them. The cause of this pattern is not known, but it has been conjectured that the nodules are denticles.

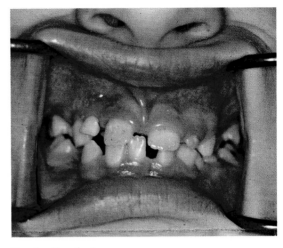

Dentin Dysplasia

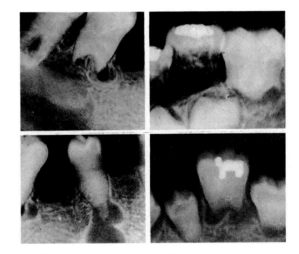

Dentin Dysplasia

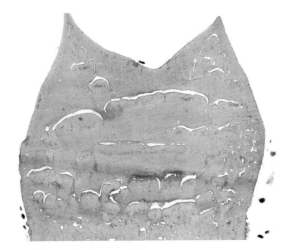

Dentin Dysplasia   × 32

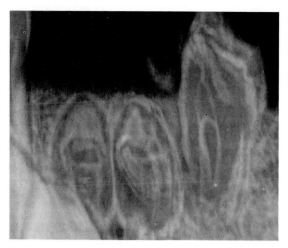

Regional Odontodysplasia

REGIONAL ODONTODYSPLASIA

(Top) This peculiar and characteristic form of odontogenic dysplasia usually involves several teeth in a quadrant or region. The teeth have a ghostlike appearance and have been termed *shell teeth.* Both dentin and enamel are affected, the dentin being sparse and poorly formed and the enamel thin and rough. The cause is unknown.

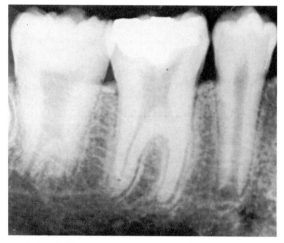

Taurodontism

TAURODONTISM

(Center) Taurodontism is an unusual dental anomaly characterized by an enlargement of the body of the tooth at the expense of the roots. The word *taurus* means bull and denotes a similarity of these teeth to those of cud-chewing or ungulate animals. The clinical shape of the crowns is normal. The condition is thought to be genetic and is widespread in most of the world's population groups. It has been observed in patients with epidermolysis bullosa and other diseases affecting tissues of ectodermal origin. It has been suggested that taurodontism may be the result of ectodermal dysplasias affecting the epithelial diaphram and Hertwig's sheath (see p. 16) but it does occur without evidence of other anomalies.

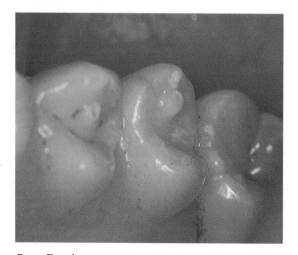

Dens Evaginatus

DENS EVAGINATUS

(Bottom) Dens evaginatus (tuberculated cusp) is a developmental anomaly occurring most often on the occlusal surface of molars and premolars. It presents clinically as a cone-shaped elevation of enamel that is frequently subjected to occlusal trauma. It probably arises as an outfolding of enamel epithelium in the early stages of odontogenesis, and contains an extension of normal pulp tissue. It is reported as being more common in persons of Mongolian racial extraction. Treatment entails removal of the tuberculated cusp, followed by pulp capping or endodontic procedures.

CLEIDOCRANIAL DYSPLASIA

This hereditary developmental disturbance is characterized primarily by defective ossification of the clavicles and bones of the skull that are not preformed in cartilage. The aplasia or hypoplasia of the clavicles enables the patient to move his shoulders forward to such an extent that he may be able to touch them together in front of the sternum. There may be a retarded closure of the fontanels and an exaggerated development of the transverse diameter of the skull. The root of the nose may be broad, the bridge depressed, and the accessory sinuses may be missing or small. Because there is usually some underdevelopment of the long bones, these individuals are frequently of relatively short stature. This disease is often associated with failure of shedding and eruption of teeth, the presence of numerous unerupted supernumerary teeth, and underdevelopment of the maxilla. This last abnormality gives a prognathic effect to the mandible. Mentality is not affected.

(Top) Cleidocranial dysplasia (Marie and Sainton's disease) in a 24-year-old male, showing the characteristic excessive mobility of the shoulders. Radiographic examination revealed defective development of the skull, clavicles, and cervical spine, as well as the presence of numerous unerupted permanent and supernumerary teeth. The patient is short, stocky, and broad-shouldered. The nose is broad, and the maxilla underdeveloped.

(Center) Cleidocranial dysplasia in a 14-year-old male. Only the mandibular permanent teeth have erupted. Delayed exfoliation of primary teeth also occurs.

(Bottom) Radiographs of a patient with a cleidocranial dysplasia, illustrating dilaceration and failure of exfoliation and eruption. Extraction of deciduous teeth usually does not aid the eruption of the permanent ones. When a prosthesis is contemplated, it is acceptable practice to leave the numerous deeply unerupted teeth in place if it appears that their removal would result in excessive bone loss. In all cases of multiple unerupted teeth, the clavicles should be examined radiographically.

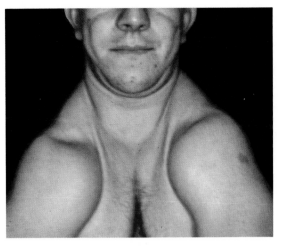

Cleidocranial Dysplasia, Excessive Shoulder Mobility

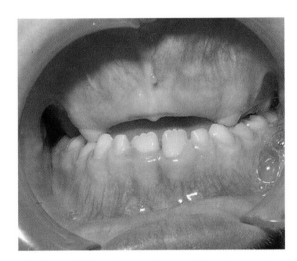

Cleidocranial Dysplasia, Retarded Eruption

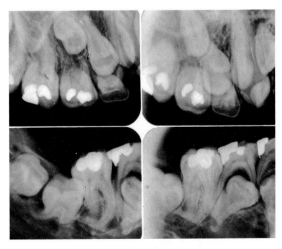

Cleidocranial Dysplasia, Unerupted Teeth

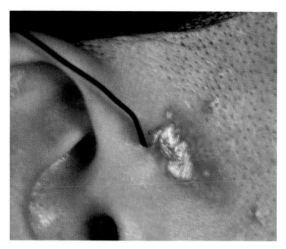

Preauricular Sinus

PREAURICULAR SINUS

(Top)   A sinus just anterior to the external ear is identified by a probe. The scar tissue resulted from a previous infection of the tract. Cysts and sinuses in this area are due to defective closure of the 1st branchial cleft. Pits found in the pinna of the ear probably are the result of faulty coalescence of the six nodules from which the auricle originates.

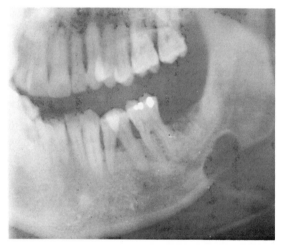

Mandibular Salivary Gland Defect

LINGUAL MANDIBULAR SALIVARY GLAND DEPRESSION

(Center)   Radiographic appearance of defect along inferior cortex of mandible in molar area. The area consists of a depression in the lingual cortex of the mandible in which a lobule of the submandibular gland is positioned. In some instances there may be actual enclavement of salivary gland tissue surrounded by bone. Similar lesions have been reported in the premolar area and incisor area of the mandible. Treatment is not necessary, although definitive diagnosis sometimes cannot be made without surgical exploration.

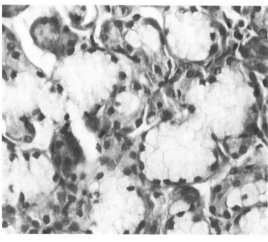

Mandibular Salivary Gland Defect   ×40

(Bottom)   Microscopic appearance of tissue removed from mandibular salivary gland defect. Pattern is identical to that of the submandibular gland (see p. 4).

Diseases of the Teeth and Supporting Structures

INTRODUCTION

Diseases of the teeth and supporting structures may be classified according to etiology, but for purposes of this Atlas it is much easier and more convenient to divide them according to the tissues involved: (1) diseases of the calcified portions of the teeth, (2) diseases of the pulp and their sequelae, and (3) diseases of the periodontium.

The calcified portions of the teeth may be worn away by the abrasive action of numerous foreign substances or by abnormal masticatory forces. Noncarious loss of tooth substance may also be due to erosion. Teeth may be stained extrinsically by such substances as chromogenic bacteria, food, drugs, and tobacco, or intrinsically during development by circulating pigments. A "pink tooth" may result from internal resorption of the dentin. Resorption of the apical portion of a permanent tooth root may be caused by improper tooth movement, endocrine imbalance, Paget's disease, neoplasia, inflammation, or may be idiopathic.

Dental caries remains the most common and important disease process affecting the hard structures of the teeth. The disease is related to the composition, form, and position of the teeth; to certain characteristics of the saliva; and to the diet, in particular the carbohydrates and possibly the phosphates. It is generally agreed that the lesions of caries begin with decalcification and that acidogenic bacteria in the dentobacterial plaque are essential to the process. Although dental caries is initiated by bacterial action, it is not an infection in the usual sense, for the tissue is not invaded by bacteria or their toxins, and the tissues that are injured (enamel and dentin) are incapable of inflammatory response.

The pulp has great recuperative powers and will recover from injuries provided that the causative agent is not too pronounced or long-acting. This tissue protects itself by the formation of reparative dentin in response to abrasion, erosion, attrition, cavity preparation, and dental caries. Under certain conditions it will heal even when exposed. The pulp and periodontal ligament have the ability to repair a root fracture.

When the pulp is severely injured by thermal changes, trauma, microorganisms, or chemical agents, the resulting pulpitis may not be resolved. If such is the case, inflammation of the periapical tissues will eventually occur if proper endodontic therapy is not instituted. Injury of the tissue in the periapical region by irritants emanating from the pulp canal may result in formation of a granuloma (chronic periapical granuloma). A granuloma may in time form a periodontal (radicular, periapical) cyst. A localized collection of pus (abscess) at the periapex may also be a sequela of pulpitis. Pus from a periapical abscess may burrow through the bone to the gingiva, forming a parulis (gingival abscess, "gum boil"). This gingival lesion may rupture, and a draining sinus may develop. Periapical infections may sometimes spread and involve the various fascial spaces of the head and neck.

Diseases of the periodontium are in general inflammatory. Gingivitis is usually initiated by local factors but may be modified by systemic factors. Bacteria are involved in most gingivitis. Occasionally blastomatoid enlargements occur from long-standing irritation of the gingiva. Periodontitis is usually preceded by gingivitis. Trauma from occlusion and systemic factors may contribute to periodontal disease, but *per se* they do not initiate periodontitis.

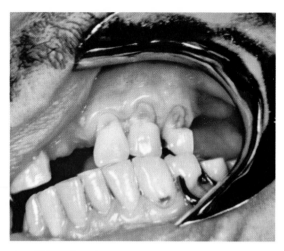

Dentifrice Abrasion

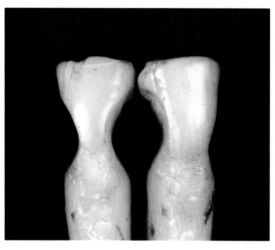

Toothpick Abrasion

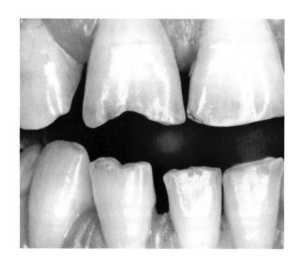

Bobby-Pin Abrasion

ABRASION

The term *abrasion* is commonly used to designate defects in tooth tissues resulting from the abrasive action of substances other than food. Abnormal tooth wear may result from improper oral hygiene procedures, from holding objects with the teeth, and from chewing on various foreign substances.

(Top) Sharp wedge-shaped defects on the maxillary left lateral, canine, and 1st premolar teeth, caused by the abrasive action of a dentifrice. Less severe dentifrice abrasion of this type may be observed frequently on the root surfaces in adults in whom gingival recession has exposed the cementum. While overzealous and improper brushing contributes to this form of abrasion, toothbrush bristles alone will not cause the defects. If enamel is involved, it is only by undermining, for modern dentifrices are not abrasive enough to wear away enamel. The canines are involved more frequently than any other teeth, owing to their prominence. The defects may be more marked on the left side of the mouth in right-handed people, and vice versa.

(Center) The misuse of toothpicks, dental floss, and dental tape may cause abnormal tooth wear. The substantial loss of tooth substance seen in the illustration was caused by the pernicious habit of rotating a toothpick between the lower central incisor teeth. Strenuously polishing the teeth with dental floss or tape apical to the cementoenamel junction may result in the notching of the root surfaces. This notching is more likely to occur when the floss or tape is used in conjunction with a dentifrice.

(Bottom) The notches in the incisal edges of the maxillary right central and mandibular right lateral were produced by using these teeth repeatedly to open bobby pins. Similar defects, though of lesser magnitude, may be produced by thread-biting. Continually holding tacks, nails, pins, or other hard substances in the teeth may also result in abnormal incisal wear. Large notches involving several teeth are sometimes observed in individuals who habitually hold a pipe in one location, especially if the stem is made of clay.

(Top) Excessive wearing of the crowns of teeth is observed most frequently in habitual tobacco chewers. The greatest amount of damage is usually seen in the lingual cusps of the maxillary teeth and the buccal cusps of the mandibular teeth. The pattern of wear, however, may vary with the habits of the patient. In some instances the abrasion may be limited to one side, and in others the entire dental arch may be involved. The loss of tooth substance in tobacco chewers is also accompanied by staining of the exposed dentin. At times the teeth may be worn to the gingival margin without exposure of dental pulps. This is possible because the pulp responds with progressive formation of reparative dentin.

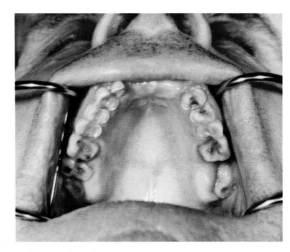

Tobacco Abrasion

(Center) Marked abrasion of the anterior teeth resulting from the chewing of betel nuts. Ordinarily these teeth are stained a dark mahogany red, but in the case illustrated prophylaxis was given so that the pattern of wear could be better demonstrated. The so-called betel nut is the fruit of the areca palm. It is commonly chewed for medicinal purposes by natives of southern India, Sri Lanka, Malaya, Thailand, Taiwan, Guam, the Philippines, and several of the small South Pacific islands. The amount of abnormal tooth wear associated with the use of the nut depends partly on the manner in which it is prepared for chewing. It may be chewed with or without the husk, but is often cut into pieces and each piece wrapped in a leaf of the betel vine with a small amount of ground sea shells or powdered coral.

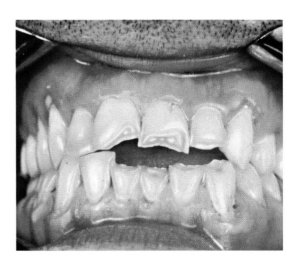

Betel-Nut Abrasion

(Bottom) Severe abrasion in a sand blaster. Fine particles of sand suspended in dust entered this patient's mouth during inspiration and resulted in the excessive wearing away of the occlusal and incisal tooth surfaces when the individual brought his teeth together into occlusion. The presence of the abrasive material in the mouth probably caused the patient to grit his teeth subconsciously, thus increasing the wear. The sharp edges of enamel resulting from occlusal and incisal abrasion from any cause may irritate the lingual, buccal, and labial mucosa and should be eliminated either by careful rounding or by restorative procedures. Sand blasters should use protective masks.

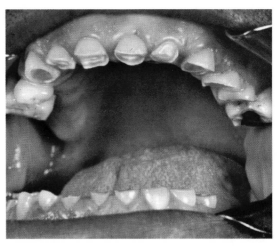

Sand Abrasion

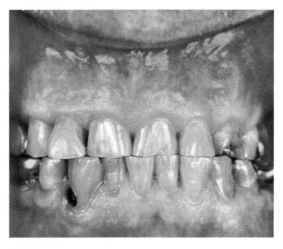

Attrition

ATTRITION

(Top)   Attrition and abrasion are not synonymous. Attrition is the physiologic wearing away of the teeth during mastication, while abrasion refers to any other type of mechanical wear. Attrition always involves functional surfaces and may be excessive due to bruxism (night grinding), gritty food, premature contacts (centric or eccentric), or abnormal tooth structures (see pp. 41, 45, and 46). Excessive wear at contact points may occur in conjunction with excessive and incisal attrition resulting in accentuation of the physiologic mesial drift of the teeth. The pulp is protected from exposure in severe cases by the formation of reparative dentin.

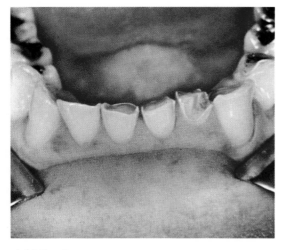

Acid Erosion

EROSION

(Center)   The use of acid in the treatment of gastric disease and the repeated regurgitation of gastric contents, as may occur in bulimia (anorexia nervosa), may result in acid erosion of the teeth. Although the saliva tends to buffer the acid, the concentration may be too high in certain areas for neutralization to occur. The acid may cause the decalcification of enamel in the regions it first touches, as seen here in a patient who took dilute hydrochloric acid from a glass tumbler. The deleterious effect of this type of therapy may be alleviated by immediate use of baking soda as a mouthwash. Once the dentin has been exposed by acid action, it may wear down rapidly, and the enamel may chip even after the acid is eliminated. People who habitually use lemons may exhibit acid erosion—usually on the labial surfaces of the anterior teeth if they suck on the fruit, and on the lingual surfaces if they chew it.

(Bottom)   Noncarious dissolution of labial and buccal enamel of unknown cause is commonly classified as idiopathic erosion. The lesions observed in this type of erosion are frequently saucer-shaped but may also be flattened, wedge-shaped or very irregular. They are differentiated from dentrifice abrasion because they originate in the enamel rather than on the root surface. After the dentin is exposed, however, these lesions may be deepened as a result of dentrifice abrasion.

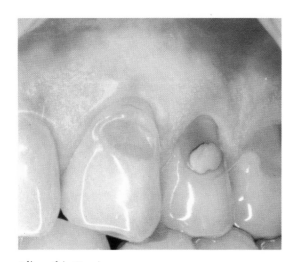

Idiopathic Erosion

STAINS

Those stains that come from within the tooth are called intrinsic stains. The most common example is discoloration of the crown by blood pigments that enter the dentinal tubules after pulpal injury. During tooth development generalized intrinsic staining may result from pigments associated with systemic disease or medications. More frequently, stains are caused by the accumulation of material on the tooth surface. These are extrinsic stains, and the color depends on the substance responsible, *e.g.*, tobacco, drugs, foods, microorganisms, and blood from the gingival crevice. Extrinsic stains may be associated with soft deposits or with calculus.

(Top) This 4-year-old child shows dark greenish-blue intrinsic pigmentation of the deciduous teeth. The child became jaundiced shortly after birth as the result of erythroblastosis fetalis. Greenish-yellow skin color was intense during the first 10 wks of life; by the 27th wk the icterus had completely disappeared. Circulating pigments caused staining of the dental tissues that were developing during the first 3 mos of life. The pigmentation is primarily in the dentin. Intrinsic staining also may occur in congenital porphyria (red-brown) or with tetracyclines (yellow-brown).

(Center) Tetracyclines and their derivatives administered during tooth development are incorporated into dentin and enamel. The teeth fluoresce in ultraviolet light. The ground section shown is a deciduous incisor from a 5 1/2-year-old girl who received oxytetracycline intermittently for 4 to 7 days at a time between the 5th and 15th mo of life. In ultraviolet light the tetracycline-affected bands have a brilliant yellow color.

(Bottom) Brown pellicle is found on the teeth of some individuals who do not use an abrasive-containing dentifrice. The pellicle may vary in thickness and coloration. This brown-stained, structureless film may be readily removed and its recurrence prevented by appropriate oral hygiene procedures. In this case the pellicle varies from very heavy on the upper centrals to mild on lower right canine. Children with poor oral hygiene may show green stain with a similar distribution.

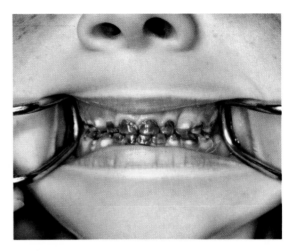

Intrinsic Stain, Bilirubin

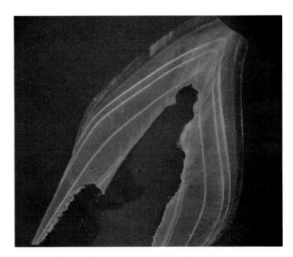

Tetracycline Fluorescence, Ground Section

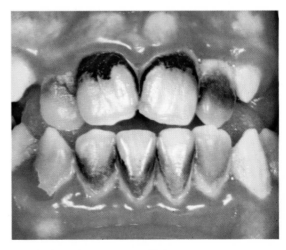

Extrinsic Stain, Brown Pellicle

ROOT FRACTURES

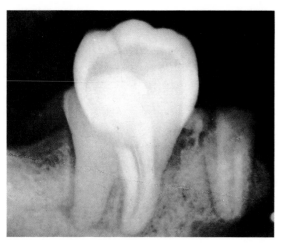

Fractured Molar Tooth

Root fractures are not common, but because of their possibility, periapical radiographs should always be taken following traumatic incidents. When the fracture line is apical to the dentogingival attachment, healing may occur, especially if the crown segment is immobilized. A fractured root heals in somewhat the same manner as an osseous fracture. There is an ingrowth of vascular fibrous connective tissue from the pulp and periodontal ligament, and subsequently the dentin surfaces resorb. Later calcified material is deposited. This material varies with the case and may be tubular or atubular dentin, bone, or cementum. In some instances the calcific continuity of the root is reestablished. In other cases a small amount of fibrous connective tissue may remain separating the tooth segments, and thus a fibrous union or pseudoarthrosis is the final result. Reducing the possibility of secondary infection by keeping the neck of the involved tooth clean, applying mild antiseptics to the gingival crevice, and using antibiotics systemically may aid materially in the successful healing of a fractured root.

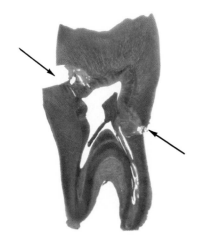

Healed Fracture   × 3

(Top)   This molar tooth was fractured by a rocket shell fragment. Even though the two portions of the tooth are not aligned properly, healing occurred. The tooth was removed 14 months after injury in order to accommodate a prosthesis. At the time of removal this tooth reacted normally to pulp tests.

(Center)   Low-power photomicrograph of the same tooth. The line of fracture is indicated by the arrows. The calcified material uniting the fractures is evident. Most of the pulp tissue was lost in the processing of the specimen.

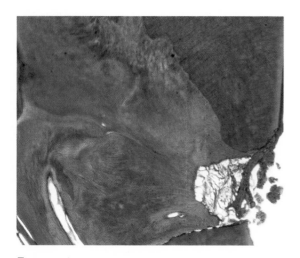

Fracture Area   × 40

(Bottom)   A higher magnification of the healed area on the right side of the same tooth shows the bonelike structure of the repairing tissue contrasted with the blue-staining tubular dentin above and below. Small scalloped regions in the dentin indicate that some resorption preceded the process of osteoid formation. The small clear area at the right has not repaired completely. It is probable that some of the calcified material associated with the healing was formed by the pulp, and other portions by the periodontal ligament.

INTERNAL RESORPTION

In this condition (also termed "idiopathic resorption") the pulp tissue undergoes a metamorphosis, resulting in resorption of the dentin from the pulpal walls. The pulp cavity in such cases, rather than being occupied by loose, delicate connective tissue that is bordered by odontoblasts, is devoid of the latter cells and filled with very vascular granulation tissue. A history of trauma may sometimes be elicited, but in most instances no cause for this phenomenon can be determined. If the process of resorption reaches the enamel, a pink spot may be seen in the crown because the highly vascular granulation tissue shows through the translucent enamel. Internal resorption ceases at times, and bonelike tissue is deposited both in the resorbed areas and haphazardly throughout the pulp. Dentin resorption usually begins from the inside, although in some instances it may be initiated from the periodontal ligament. Technically, the latter type is classified as external resorption. In cases in which there is perforation of the root it is not always clear whether internal or external resorption has occurred.

(Top) Internal resorption as seen radiographically in a maxillary 2nd molar tooth. While most of the crown and a portion of the distal root are radiolucent, it is apparent that some osteoid formation has already occurred.

(Center) In this cross section of the tooth shown above, loss of purple-staining dentin from the pulpal wall is evident. It is also apparent that osteoid (red-stained) has replaced some of the lost dentin, and that trabeculae have developed in the pulp. The presence of the trabeculae probably accounts for the somewhat mottled appearance in the radiograph.

(Bottom) A higher magnification of one of the trabeculae extending from the pulpal wall shows tubular dentin surrounded by osteoid or osteodentin. A line of osteoblasts is seen in the baylike area along the upper left portion of the spicule. Inflammatory cells are apparent in the fibrous pulp tissue.

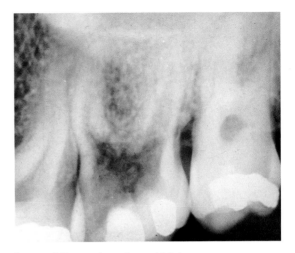

Internal Resorption, Second Molar

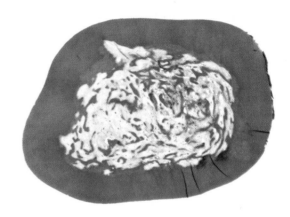

Internal Resorption, Cross Section ×6

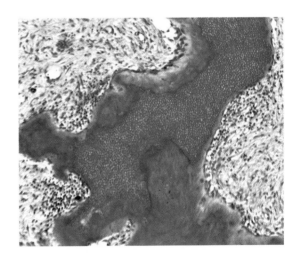

Internal Resorption, Same Specimen as Above ×100

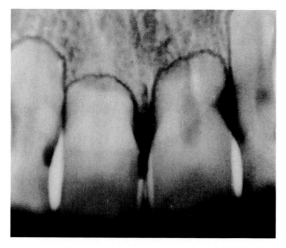

Apical Resorption, Maxillary Anterior Teeth

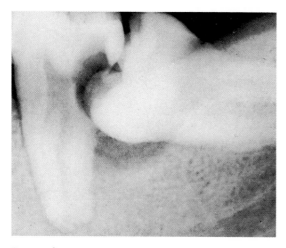

External Resorption

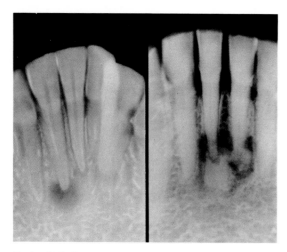

*Periapical Cementum Dysplasia, Early and
Advanced Stages*

EXTERNAL RESORPTION

(Top) Apical resorption may occur following orthodontic treatment, as a result of endocrine imbalance (particularly hypothyroidism), in association with Paget's disease, or no precise cause may be evident. In the normal individual receiving proper orthodontic therapy, no gross resorption should be expected. The patient's history is of great importance in determining the cause of any given resorption. Inflammation, especially suppurative, in the periapical region may cause root resorption, but the resorbed areas are not replaced by bone. Malignant neoplasm, either local or metastatic, may cause root resorption (see pp. 166, 180). Apical resorption should be differentiated from underdeveloped roots (see pp. 37, 104). Histological examination of teeth frequently reveals small areas of resorption not demonstrated radiographically.

(Center) External resorption of a mandibular 2nd molar in association with an impacted 3rd molar. Eruption-type pressure from the 3rd molar probably activated osteoclasts of the periodontal ligament, and these then resorbed the cementum and dentin of the 2nd molar root.

PERIAPICAL CEMENTUM DYSPLASIA

(Bottom) This lesion, variously termed periapical cementoma, benign periapical fibroma, focal fibro-osseous dysplasia, and traumatic osteoclasia as well as periapical cementum dysplasia, usually appears at the apical region of mandibular incisor teeth with healthy pulps. In its early stage, a radiolucency appears (first stage cementoma) that is gradually replaced by radiopaque material, which may be cementum or sclerotic bone. It has been suggested that occlusal trauma may contribute to the development of these lesions, but the evidence is inconclusive. In general, surgical intervention is not indicated for these nonneoplastic lesions.

DENTAL CARIES

Dental caries is initiated by decalcification beginning at the tooth surfaces. It is generally accepted that the decalcifying acids are produced in the dentobacterial plaques by the action of bacteria on carbohydrates. The dentobacterial plaques are found on protected areas of the teeth that are not kept clean by the action of the tongue, lips, cheeks, the food bolus, or oral hygiene. Carious lesions, therefore, most frequently occur in the occlusal fissures, interproximally or cervically. A few individuals are resistant to caries regardless of their carbohydrate intake. Optimal amounts of fluorides ingested in the water during tooth development will lower the incidence of dental caries.

(Top)   The initial lesion of dental caries, clinically, is a white spot, which may become stained. Histologically, the appearance of such a lesion, on the interproximal surfaces, is a cone-shaped region of decalcification with its broad base at the surface. In the section shown there are two such cone-shaped lesions extending toward the dentinoenamel junction. At one point along the surface some enamel has disintegrated. A sharp explorer might be expected to reveal this defect.

(Center)   In this section the carious process has extended into the dentin, but there still is no cavitation. There is broad involvement of the enamel surface, and the apex of the cone of decalcification has reached the dentinoenamel junction. Here the process spreads laterally, and a cone of decalcification in the dentin is stained red. A surrounding halo of white suggests that the dentinal calcification has increased (sclerosis) as a defense against the advance of caries. Clinically this lesion would be radiolucent.

(Bottom)   This section shows frank cavitation, presumably due to disintegration of the decalcified enamel. The overhanging enamel could easily be fractured during mastication or by an operative hand instrument. The carious process is advancing within the dentin as indicated by the red-stained area and the reactive region beneath.

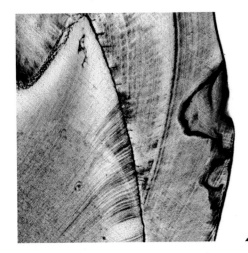

Interproximal Caries, Early Enamel Lesion, Ground Section

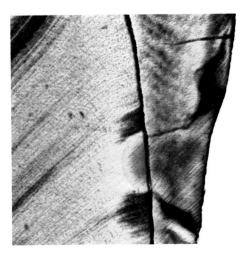

Interproximal Caries Involving Enamel and Dentin, Ground Section

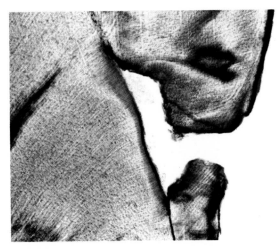

Interproximal Caries with Cavitation, Ground Section

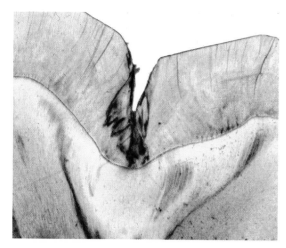

Fissural Caries, Ground Section

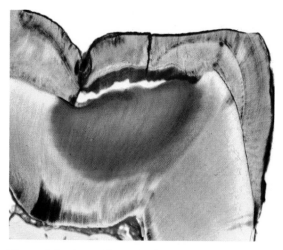

Fissural Caries with Marked Dentinal Involvement, Ground Section

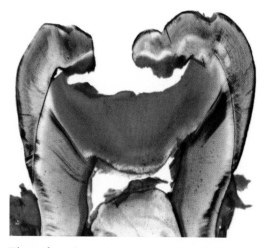

Fissural Caries, Advanced with Cavitation, Ground Section

DENTAL CARIES *(continued)*

Dental caries beginning in pits and fissures presents a somewhat different pattern in its advance through the enamel from that of smooth-surface caries although the chemical and physical processes involved probably are identical. As the process of caries follows the direction of the enamel rods, it diverges from the enamel surface of the fissure or pit, spreading as it advances toward the dentin. This results in a cone-shaped lesion with its base toward or at the dentinoenamel junction. Even though there may be extensive destruction of the underlying enamel and dentin *(center)*, the site of initiation of caries usually remains small, and the patient may be unaware of the lesion until pulpal involvement causes pain or until the roof of the enamel over the cavity collapses under masticatory forces. A small opening leading to a large carious lesion may be overlooked during a screening or cursory clinical examination. The use of pit and fissure sealants prior to clinical evidence of caries is a recommended procedure.

(Top)   Caries is seen beginning in a fissure with decalcification extending from its sides and bottom. If this process had continued, a greater area would be involved at the dentinoenamel junction than at the surface as indicated by the width of the pale yellow lesion in the dentin.

(Center)   When occlusal caries reaches the dentin, it usually spreads laterally as seen here. There may be separation of the enamel from the dentin and later fracture of the enamel "roof." The red-staining regions of enamel and dentin are zones of decalcification. The process of decalcification of enamel from the underlying dentin (red region above separation) is known as undermining, secondary, or backward caries of the enamel. A zone of increased calcification (sclerosis) surrounds the red zone of decalcification in the dentin, but not in the enamel, which has no such defense mechanism.

(Bottom)   In this section the caries is far advanced, and the red-staining zone appears to have reached the pulpal wall. The process of cavitation has left overhanging enamel which could be fractured easily. At this stage the pulp would be involved and the patient would experience pain (odontalgia).

When sections are decalcified in the laboratory, all the enamel except the organic portion (matrix and lamellae) is lost, and even this portion is lost unless special technics are used. The dentin, having a greater organic content (about 30% vs. 2% for enamel), is well preserved after histologic preparation.

(Top) The light-lavender-staining material above is enamel matrix in a decalcified section. A lamella is seen as a darker-staining, curved structure extending through the matrix. The dark-staining granules in the red-stained dentin are microorganisms in dentinal tubules.

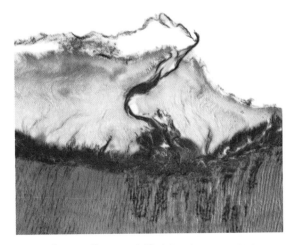

Enamel Lamella, Decalcified Section ×200

(Center) Caries in the dentin. A small dentobacterial plaque is present on the surface. The carious process follows the dentinal tubules. The inorganic portion of the dentin probably is first decalcified by bacterially produced acids. Because of its higher inorganic content the dentin is not extensively dissolved, and its morphology is not altered by the decalcification. When proteolytic activity is combined with or follows decalcification, the dentin is completely disintegrated. The dark streaks in the photomicrograph are enlarged tubules containing microorganisms. At various places along the bacteria-packed tubules beadlike enlargements are seen. These distentions (liquefaction foci) are assumed to result from the pressure of bacterial growth after the dentinal matrix is softened by decalcification. They enlarge by proteolysis and coalescence.

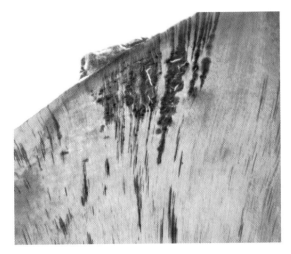

Dentinal Caries, Decalcified Section ×35

(Bottom) A higher magnification of the specimen above shows details of the dentobacterial plaque at the surface with the raylike arrangement of some of its organisms. Filaments (actinomycetes), bacilli, and cocci commonly make up this plaque, which sometimes is erroneously called the mucin plaque. In the dentin the details of the microorganisms in the tubules and the liquefaction foci, with cracks where the entire dentinal substance has been lost, are apparent. The bacteria may extend into tubules in advance of the process of decalcification and may even infect the pulp while the dentin is intact.

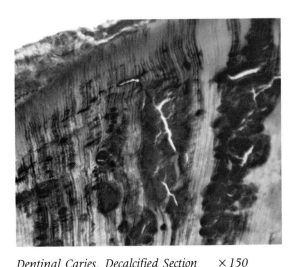

Dentinal Caries, Decalcified Section ×150

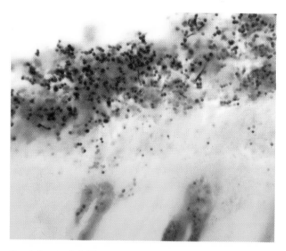

Dentobacterial Plaque, Brown and Brenn Stain, Decalcified Section ×918

DENTAL CARIES *(continued)*

(Top) This dentobacterial plaque is stained to show some of the microorganisms. Dentobacterial plaques are masses of different species of microorganisms. The filaments appear to form the basic structure, clinging tenaciously to the tooth surface. Many of the acidogenic organisms in the plaque rapidly convert carbohydrate into acid. Other bacteria produce proteolytic enzymes that dissolve the organic materials of the tooth. Plaques are difficult to remove by ordinary oral hygienic procedures and reform rapidly after removal. Antibacterial agents in dentifrices or mouth washes may augment the mechanical removal of plaque.

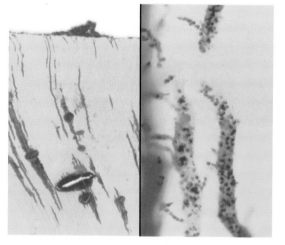

×85 *Dentinal Caries* ×920
Brown and Brenn Stain, Decalcified Sections

(Center) In the left photomicrograph there is plaque on the surface of the dentin, and bacteria have penetrated along the tubules. Foci of liquefaction are also apparent. The right photomicrograph shows microorganisms in enlarged dentinal tubules. A few are extending out into the lateral branches. The bacteria may progress along the tubules to the pulp or destroy the surrounding dentin by decalcification and proteolysis.

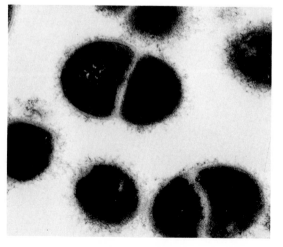

Streptococcus mutans ×27,000

(Bottom) The essential role of bacteria in initiation of caries has been demonstrated. The most cariogenic organism has proved to be *Streptococcus mutans.* This organism initially adheres to a tooth surface by a specific molecular configuration on the cell wall. It has the ability to form lactic, formic, and other acids rapidly from sucrose and glucose, and the ability to survive in a low-*p*H environment. Some species of *Lactobacillus* and *Actinomyces* appear to be associated with some forms of dental caries.

The generally accepted methods for control of dental caries are plaque removal by brushing and flossing, as part of a home care program; reducing the frequency of intake of refined carbohydrates; fluoridation of water supplies and topical application of fluorides by approved techniques including fluoridated dentrifices; and use of pit and fissure sealants.

SECONDARY AND REPARATIVE DENTIN

(Top) Secondary dentin as a protective layer is formed on the pulpal wall continuously throughout life. Reparative dentin is formed as a result of dental caries, cavity preparation, abrasion, attrition, or erosion. Stimulation of odontoblastic processes accelerates this dentin formation in the region of the involved odontoblasts. This is exemplified in the photomicrograph, which shows a cavity preparation at the right and a slight excess of red-staining reparative dentin along the pulpal wall. If the course of the dentinal tubules is traced from the axial cavity wall to the pulp, it will be seen that this reparative dentin has been formed at the pulpal ends of the cut tubules. Secondary dentin is present on the opposite side of the pulp chamber.

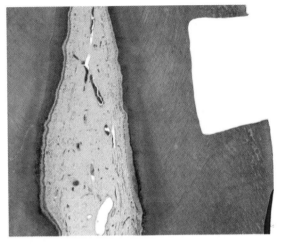

Reparative Dentin Beneath Cavity Preparation × 15

PULP HEALING

Pulp capping has been practiced for many years, and claims have been made in favor of various drugs and techniques for this procedure. For the most part these claims have been based on clinical evidence alone. However, necrosis of the pulp may occur, or a mild chronic inflammation exist, without symptoms. In general, the success of a pulp-capping operation should be based on histologic evidence. Therefore only those procedures should be used which have been proved by laboratory studies to be consistently followed by complete pulp healing.

(Center) Successful pulp capping in a human tooth. At lower left is normal pulp tissue covered by a bridge of dentin. In this case the pulp was deliberately exposed and the wound covered with a paste of calcium hydroxide and tap water. The tooth, which needed to be removed for orthodontic purposes, was extracted 10 wk after the pulp-capping procedure.

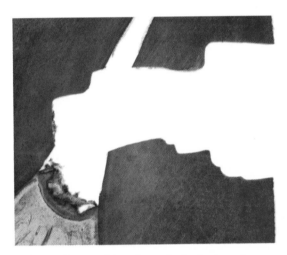

Pulp Healing, Bridge of Dentin in Region of Exposure × 20

(Bottom) Photomicrograph of another section from the tooth shown in the center picture. At the base of the newly formed tubular dentin is a row of well-differentiated odontoblasts. The underlying pulp is vital, quite cellular, and free of inflammatory elements.

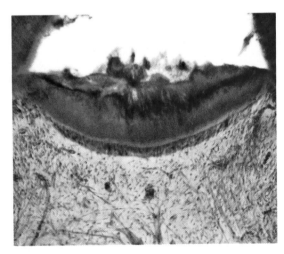

Pulp Healing, Bridge of Dentin, Normal Pulp × 100

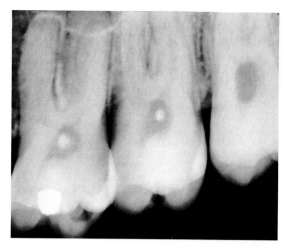

Denticles in Coronal Pulp of First and Second Molars

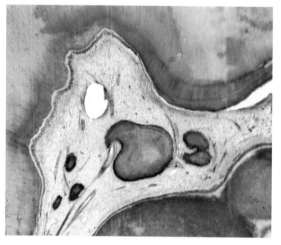

Denticles in Coronal Pulp of Molar Tooth   × 18

PULP CALCIFICATION

Calcifications in the pulp may appear as roughly circular areas (denticles, pulp stones, pulp nodules) or as diffuse, irregular deposits. Denticles may be attached to the wall of the pulp or may be free within the pulp cavity. True denticles are composed of tubular dentin, but most pulp stones are lamellar structures with few, if any, tubules. Non-tubular denticles are termed false pulp stones.

(Top)   Radiopaque areas (pulp stones) are apparent in the coronal pulps of the maxillary 1st and 2nd molars. These denticles are distinct, but frequently they are only faintly discernible, and many pulp stones that could not be demonstrated radiographically can be found in histologic sections. Some individuals show pulp stones in nearly every tooth. Referred pain is sometimes attributed to pressure of pulp stones on nerves, but removal of teeth with pulp stones and no other symptoms seldom eliminates neuralgic pain. Caution is important, and hasty decisions to extract such teeth as possible causes of pain should be avoided.

(Center)   One large denticle and several small ones lying free in the coronal pulp of a molar tooth that was symptomless but was removed to accommodate a prosthetic appliance. None of these pulp stones is composed of tubular dentin. It is apparent that the largest one has been formed in concentric layers. No inflammatory cells are present, and, except for the calcific deposits, the pulp is normal. Pulpal calcifications are a common histologic finding and are probably present in about 80% of adult teeth. Many of these denticles are quite small, however, and are not apparent radiographically.

(Bottom)   The irregular, purplish-staining areas in the central portion of this photomicrograph are regions of diffuse calcification. Incomplete tissue fixation is evident from the lack of odontoblasts and the general character of the tissue. There is a tendency for calcium salts to be deposited in the pulp, as elsewhere in the body, in tissue that is necrotic or degenerating. Diffuse, linear, dystrophic calcification in the pulp is generally limited to the radicular portion and is observed most frequently in older individuals.

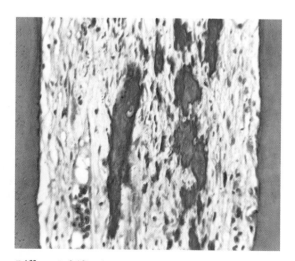

Diffuse Calcification   × 35

PULPITIS

(Top) Hyperemia, as shown in the radicular pulp of this tooth, is the earliest stage of inflammation. It may occur in the pulp following an operative procedure and resolve in a short period of time without the passage of leukocytes through capillary walls. This might account for some sensitivity subsequent to operative procedures, which then disappears.

In inflammation, hyperemia is followed quickly by the exudation of the fluid and cellular elements of the blood. This exudate is of a higher specific gravity than the transudate of noninflammatory edema. Exudation occurs as the result of vasodilation, increased permeability of vessel walls, and elevation of capillary pressure. It is believed that certain factors liberated by injured cells are responsible for initiating some of the vascular changes as well as directly attracting the neutrophils to the area of injury.

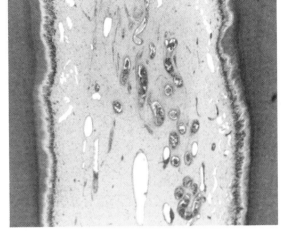

Hyperemia   × 40

(Center) A small focus of lymphocytes and plasma cells is seen in the vicinity of nerve tissue. Pulpitis, like inflammation in other tissues, is a response of the pulp to an irritant that is intense enough to injure cells. Pulpal cells may be injured or killed by microorganisms, by toxic substances, by excessive thermal change, and by trauma. Occasionally, pulpitis occurs secondarily by extension of periodontal inflammation or as a result of bacteremia (anachoretic pulpitis).

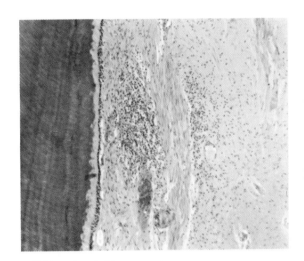

Mild Focal Pulpitis   × 98

(Bottom) A large occlusal carious area in a molar tooth is apparent at the top of the photomicrograph. In relation to this area, at the periphery of the pulp, is a thick layer of predentin. Numerous capillaries in the pulp are dilated, and in the pulpal horn there is extensive hemorrhage and a marked influx of inflammatory cells. The spaces at the left are artifacts produced in preparation of the specimen.

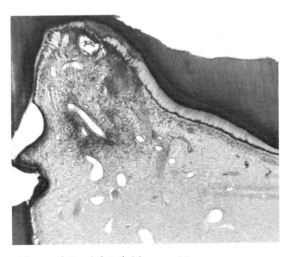

Advanced Partial Pulpitis   × 35

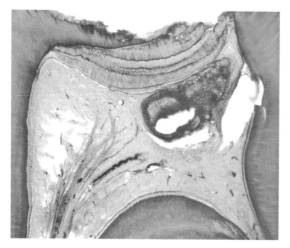

Acute Pulpal Abscess × 22

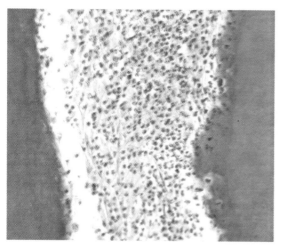

Total Suppurative Pulpitis × 190

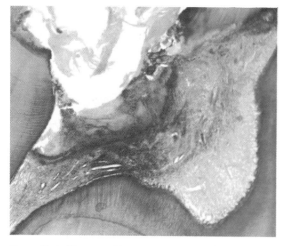

Open Pulpitis × 23

PULPITIS *(continued)*

(Top) Histologic examination of this tooth, which was removed after the patient experienced 12 hr of excruciating pain, reveals a large occlusal defect, below which are several layers of reparative dentin. In the coronal portion of the pulp is a distinctly localized mass of inflammatory cells. It is composed mainly of dead and disintegrating neutrophils. The necrotic tissue in this area is beginning to liquefy. Histologically this abscess (localized collection of pus) is acute, for there is no evidence of fibrosis at its periphery.

(Center) In this instance the suppurative exudate is not localized, and the entire pulp is involved. (The photomicrograph shows only a small area of the pulp in one of the roots.) It is apparent that the pulp tissue is necrotic and that much of it is liquefied. The inflammatory cells present are mainly neutrophils. The odontoblastic layer has been destroyed and a few neutrophils occupy lacunae along the right wall.

(Bottom) A large portion of the coronal pulp is exposed and open to the oral environment. In the necrotic area there are neutrophils, fibrin, and colonies of microorganisms. A bandlike bluish line, running the whole length of the defect, separates the viable from the nonviable tissue. This line is due to a peculiar diffusion of chromatin from dead cells. Below the necrotic area is an extensive infiltration of inflammatory cells which involves most of the coronal pulp.

Interest in pulpal reactions was stimulated with the introduction of operative procedures involving high-speed instruments. The studies of several investigators suggest that the pulp has greater recuperative powers than was formerly recognized, but all warn that every effort should be made to minimize operative trauma to the pulp by using an effective fluid coolant with high-speed instruments. With severe injury the pulp may not recover because its recuperative powers are limited by lack of room for swelling, and because it has no collateral blood supply.

(Top) Chronic hyperplastic pulpitis (pulp polyp) occurs only when the coronal pulp is widely exposed and an exceptionally good blood supply is available. Because of the latter requirement this lesion develops only in young individuals, especially in teeth that have large apical foramina. In the case shown there is a marked proliferation of granulation tissue extending outward to form a polypoid mass. The lower portion of the coronal pulp is relatively free of inflammatory cells. Frequently the surface of a pulp polyp becomes epithelialized. This probably happens when epithelial cells are scraped off the tongue or check by the sharp edges of the carious tooth and transplanted onto the well-vascularized granulation tissue of the polyp. In hyperplastic pulpitis the potential recuperative ability of pulp tissue is well demonstrated. It is apparent that when the pulp has a good blood supply and room to expand because of wide exposure, it will remain vital and make a valiant attempt at healing even when subjected to extensive irritation.

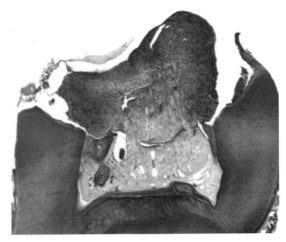

Chronic Hyperplastic Pulpitis (Pulp Polyp)   × 12

(Center) A pulp polyp in a molar of a 15-year-old patient. It extends upward almost to the line of occlusion. Because of the smooth, shiny surface it may be assumed that this polyp is covered by epithelium. Such a lesion should not be confused with hyperplastic gingival tissue that has grown into a large carious area. Pulp polyps are not particularly sensitive to touch, but they do bleed easily unless covered by epithelium.

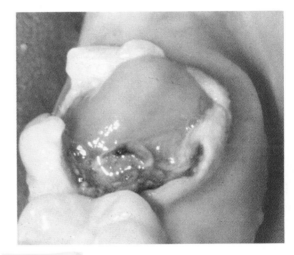

Pulp Polyp

(Bottom) Complete necrosis of the pulp in a deciduous molar tooth. Nuclear staining is absent, and the pulp chamber is filled with amorphous material and colonies of microorganisms. Total death of the pulp may result from the diffusion of chemical substances through the pulp, from thrombosis initiated by various types of total pulpitis, or from trauma severe enough to cause a loss of vascular continuity. The color of a tooth with a necrotic pulp may differ from that of adjacent normal teeth. This discoloration, which varies from yellow to gray or black, is due to staining of the dentinal tubules by pigments that are derived from the breakdown of red blood cells and the end products of protein degradation.

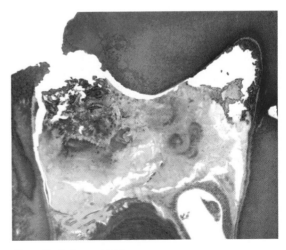

Necrotic Pulp   × 22

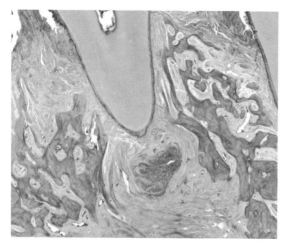

Dental Granuloma   × 8

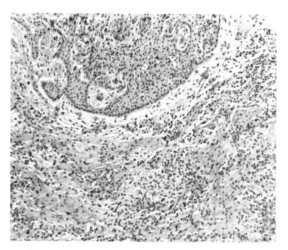

Proliferating Epithelium in Dental Granuloma
× 90

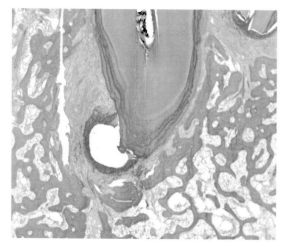

Apical Periodontal Cyst   × 8

SEQUELAE OF PULPITIS

Pulpal inflammation that is not eliminated by resolution, endodontics, or surgery usually results in periapical inflammation. This inflammatory reaction is caused most frequently by irritants emanating from the pulp although trauma also may cause periapical inflammation. The irritants from the pulp may be microorganisms, bacterially produced toxins, or products of protein degradation. Because agents other than microorganisms also cause injury, periapical inflammation may or may not be an infection. The character of the tissue response depends on the causative agent and the capacity for response of the patient's cells. Sequelae of pulpitis include dental granuloma, periodontal cyst, periapical abscess, gingival abscess, extraoral fistula, cellulitis, osteomyelitis (see p. 131), and actinomycosis (see p. 89).

(Top) Chronic productive periodontitis (dental granuloma) at apex of a premolar tooth. A large area of bone is replaced by granulation tissue in which there are numerous inflammatory cells. In such a lesion repair is taking place, but exudation continues because cells are still being injured. If the irritating factor is eliminated, healing can occur.

(Center)   If the chronic productive periodontitis involves a portion of the periodontal ligament that contains epithelial rests (see p. 16), this epithelium may be stimulated to proliferate. Such an area of epithelial proliferation is apparent at the top of this photomicrograph of a dental granuloma.

Apical Periodontal Cyst

(Bottom) An apical periodontal cyst (closed epithelium-lined space containing fluid or semifluid) forms when a mass of epithelial cells in a dental granuloma proliferates to such a degree that the central cells outgrow their vascular supply, become necrotic, and liquefy. Once a cyst has formed, periapical curettage is usually necessary in addition to proper pulp canal therapy if the periapical tissues are to regenerate. Curettage is important only in removing the epithelium-lined cyst. If a cyst is allowed to remain even after the original inflammatory irritant is eliminated, it may continue to enlarge by accumulation of fluid within the cyst and will destroy the surrounding tissue by pressure.

(Top) Two apical periodontal cysts at the apices of anterior teeth. Radiographically an apical periodontal cyst cannot be differentiated definitely from a granuloma, even though the radiolucent area is surrounded by a line of increased density. Large, circular, well-demarcated areas of decreased density, however, are suggestive of cysts.

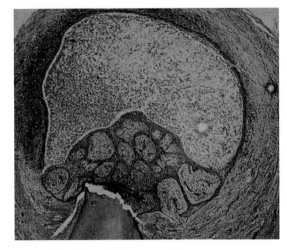

Apical Periodontal Cyst   × 12

(Center) Low-power view of an apical periodontal cyst attached to the apex of a root. The connective tissue wall of the cyst is continuous with the periodontal ligament. The epithelium that lines the cyst is squamous and arose from epithelial debris of Malassez (epithelial rests). It approximates the root in the region of the apical foramen. Epithelial rests are present in all dental granulomas, and for this reason all are potential cysts. In the region of the apex the epithelium shows proliferative changes, as is indicated by the reticular pattern. The cyst cavity is filled with tissue debris and fluid. In many instances cholesterol crystals are present in such cystic cavities and may give an oily "glare" to the cystic contents under gross examination. At times epithelial degeneration in cysts permits the contents to contact connective tissue and initiate an inflammatory response. The cyst may fill with exudate, which is sometimes purulent. No microorganisms are present. The reaction is to the toxic products of tissue degradation. The inflammatory change may be attended by pain that calls attention to the presence of the cyst.

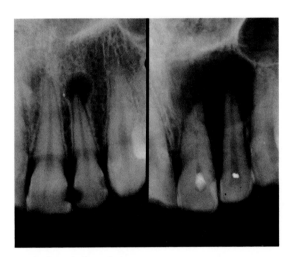

Apical Periodontal Cysts

(Bottom) Periapical radiograph of a residual cyst with a radiopaque wall. Residual cysts are remnants of periodontal cysts (or occasionally dentigerous cysts) left in the jaws following extraction of the associated teeth. They may remain asymptomatic for many years but may enlarge and produce symptoms. Radiolucencies suspected of being residual cysts should be examined by an oral pathologist to differentiate them from odontogenic keratocysts (p. 34), which may have a similar appearance.

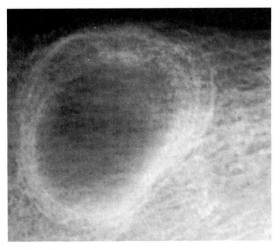

Residual Cyst

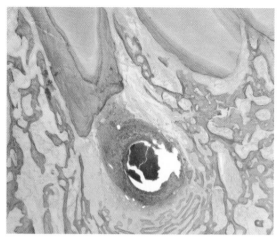

Periapical Abscess   × 8

Periapical Abscess

(Top) An abscess (localized collection of pus) in the periapical region of a premolar tooth. In the central portion of the inflammatory focus is a cavity partially filled with liquefied tissue debris and neutrophils. This type of lesion forms when an inflammatory exudate containing many neutrophils is able to confine an irritant of great intensity that has killed numerous cells. The great numbers of neutrophils liberate a large amount of a proteolytic enzyme that liquefies the necrotic tissue (both fixed tissue and dead leukocytes), forming a semi-liquid material, pus. The wall of an acute abscess is composed only of inflammatory cells, whereas fibrous tissue is found in the outer wall of a chronic abscess.

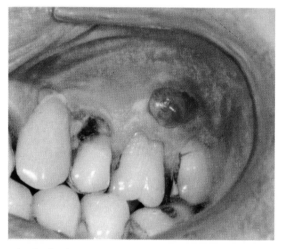

Gingival Abscess (Parulis)

(Center) The contents of the periapical abscess may be under great pressure due to an active inflammatory process forming additional pus. The pressure tends to force the pus into the surrounding tissue, and it naturally progresses along the lines of least resistance. It may burrow through the buccal cortical plate and emerge in the gingival mucosa. Accumulation of pus in this location, as shown in the illustration, is termed a *parulis,* or gingival abscess. If the pressure continues to increase, the parulis will rupture, pus will be evacuated, and the gingival swelling will regress. The evacuating tract thus formed may epithelialize, resulting in a permanent, draining sinus, or its peripheral portion may heal and a gingival abscess again develop. A parulis may also result from extension of a periodontal abscess, which is formed when pus is trapped in the wall of a narrow periodontal pocket.

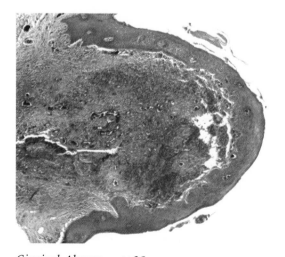

Gingival Abscess   × 28

(Bottom) Photomicrograph of a gingival abscess similar to the one seen in the center picture. In the plane of this section the covering epithelium is intact, and just below it is a mass of inflammatory cells. In one region, near the apex of the specimen, is a partially clear area containing pus. The horizontal slit extending to the left border of the picture is part of the inflammatory tract that led to the periapical lesion.

(Top)   This patient had a periapical abscess of the mandibular left 2nd molar. In this case the pus, influenced by gravity and following the line of least resistance, burrowed through the bone in a region that led to the masticatory space. Finally it extended into the subcutaneous tissue, and an abscess was formed beneath the skin. A cutaneous abscess may erupt through the skin and evacuate its purulent contents.

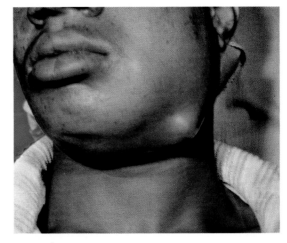

Cutaneous Abscess

(Center)   Marked swelling of the left side has resulted from extension of periapical inflammation. A diffuse nonsuppurative inflammatory process of this type is characterized by abundant serous exudation into the loose tissues. While it is commonly called "cellulitis," this is actually an edema which may resolve without suppuration, or which may progress to true cellulitis with diffuse suppuration, or in which an abscess or a phlegmon may develop.

(Bottom)   A phlegmon is an intense inflammatory process that spreads through tissue spaces over a wide area and is difficult to control. It is caused by microorganisms of high virulence and characterized by an exudate in which neutrophils predominate. Complications may arise when the spreading inflammation involves vessel walls. This causes roughening of the ordinarily smooth intima, and elements of the blood adhere to it, forming a thrombus (thrombophlebitis). Microorganisms frequently invade the vessel wall, enter the thrombus, and continue to multiply (septic thrombosis). Once the clot is infected, it tends to soften, and fragments of it may break off and enter the general circulation, causing septicemia. By this same mechanism, septic thrombosis of the cavernous sinus may occasionally occur from a periapical infection when certain veins are involved. *Ludwig's angina* is a severe phlegmonous infection in the floor of the mouth and neck. It usually is very firm and initiated by an uncontrolled odontogenic infection of the mandibular 1st molar or teeth anterior to it. The prognosis of cavernous sinus thrombosis and phlegmonous inflammation was very poor prior to the advent of antibiotic therapy. The photomicrograph is a section from the floor of the mouth in a fatal case of phlegmonous inflammation. The two dark-staining ovoid areas are veins. Inflammatory cells have invaded the vessel walls. The lumina are partially occluded by septic thrombi.

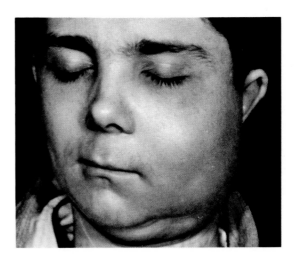

"Cellulitis"

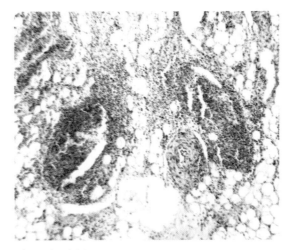

Thrombophlebitis   ×80

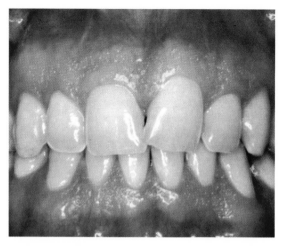

Normal Gingiva

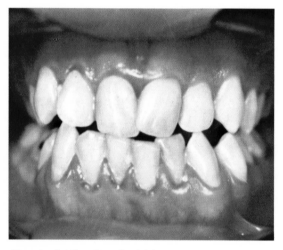

Marginal (Simple) Gingivitis

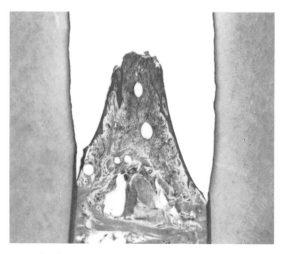

Marginal Gingivitis, Interdental Papilla ×24

NORMAL GINGIVA

The gingiva is the soft tissue surrounding the teeth and covering the adjacent alveolar process. The portion coronal to the dentogingival junction is free gingiva, while the remainder is attached gingiva. The gingival crevice or sulcus, normally not more than 2 mm in depth, is located between the tooth and the free gingiva (see p. 3). The part of the gingiva that occupies the interdental space is the interdental papilla.

(Top) Firm, healthy gingiva that is relatively normal (for age 40 years) showing characteristic sharp-edged free margins that approximate the contour of the cementoenamel junction. The pale pink, stippled gingival tissue is readily differentiated from the adjacent red vascular vestibular mucosa. The contour of the attached gingiva reflects the contour of the surface of the alveolar process.

Any survey of gingival tissue should include observations of color, form, density, and depth of the sulcus. The normal gingival color may vary from pale pink to a deep bluish-purple depending on the intensity of melanogenesis from light-colored to dark-colored individuals. Knowledge of the appearance of normal gingiva is prerequisite for recognition of the different types of periodontal disease.

MARGINAL (SIMPLE) GINGIVITIS

(Center) A mild inflammation of the free gingiva, exhibiting two of the cardinal signs of inflammation: redness (rubor) and swelling (tumor). In this case these changes, which result from congestion and exudation, are most marked in the lower anterior region and about the necks of the maxillary right central and lateral incisors.

(Bottom) The clear areas on either side of this interdental papilla were occupied by the enamel, which has been lost in preparing the specimen. The epithelium has been destroyed at the top of the papilla but still lines the sulci on either side. The large clear areas are dilated vessels and the dark-blue-staining material, most prominent near the tip, is chiefly inflammatory cells, identified under higher magnification as lymphocytes and plasma cells. The inflammation does not extend below the transseptal fibers extending between the teeth at the bottom of the picture.

(Top) A rather severe case of marginal gingivitis resulting from the irritating effect of soft and hard accretions on the teeth. There is alteration of color, form and density of the gingiva. The inflammation is most marked about the maxillary left canine and lateral incisor, where an accumulation of materia alba is evident. Lack of home care and the diminished cleansing action of food, due to irregularity of the teeth, were important etiologic factors. In marginal gingivitis the gingival sulcus is often increased in depth. In uncomplicated gingivitis this is due to gingival enlargement rather than to deepening of the gingival sulcus by apical positioning of the gingival cuff (dentogingival junction).

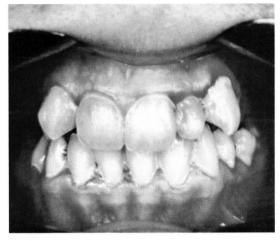

Severe Marginal Gingivitis, Before Treatment

(Center) The patient shown above after removal of soft and hard deposits and institution of proper home care. The treatment is incomplete, but marked improvement is evident. Most of the gingiva has a pale pink color and a dull, stippled surface, and the gingival margins are thinner. These changes occur rapidly after local irritants are removed, but if the disease is not treated it may progress rapidly into periodontitis.

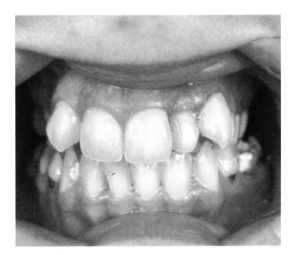

Same Case as Above, After Prophylaxis

ACUTE HERPETIC GINGIVOSTOMATITIS

(Bottom) Characteristic gingival response to primary infection by the herpes simplex virus. The primary infection, which occurs most frequently in children, is also characterized by malaise, fever, lymphadenitis, and pharyngitis. Small vesicles which may form on the gingiva in this disease are often not seen because they rapidly macerate, producing painful ulcers. The entire gingiva is intensely red, but this may go unobserved because of the presence of desquamating epithelium, which forms a grayish membranous covering. This epithelial debris can be removed easily without hemorrhage resulting, and the red color is then strikingly apparent. In the case shown there is redness at the gingival margins of some teeth, and the membrane may be observed in other areas. An herpetic ulcer is apparent in the labial mucosa (lower left foreground). (See p. 87 for recurrent herpes.)

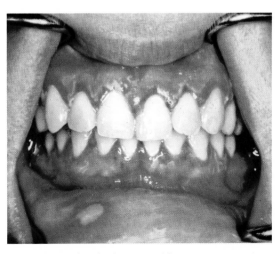

Acute Herpetic Gingivostomatitis

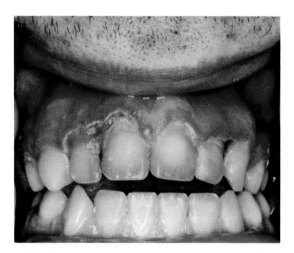

Acute Necrotizing Ulcerative Gingivitis

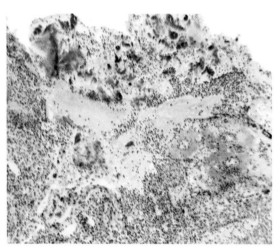

Gingival Papillae, Necrotizing Ulcerative Gingivitis
×85

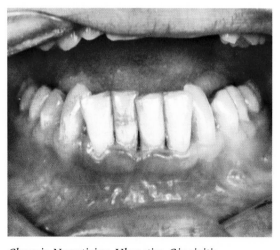

Chronic Necrotizing Ulcerative Gingivitis

NECROTIZING ULCERATIVE GINGIVITIS

(VINCENT'S INFECTION)

Necrotizing ulcerative gingivitis (ulceromembranous gingivitis, Vincent's infection, or trench mouth) is a noncommunicable inflammatory disease of the gingiva resulting from local irritation and the effects from fusiforms and spirochetes. The organisms, which are components of the normal oral flora, invade the gingival tissue when its resistance is lowered.

(Top) The acute phase of the disease is characterized by redness, swelling, ulceration, bleeding, and pain. The grayish pseudomembrane that usually covers the ulcerated surface can easily be removed, leaving a raw, bleeding base. The ulceration is often limited to the interdental area but may extend onto the labial or lingual gingiva about the necks of the teeth. The disease is also seen frequently in the region of partially erupted 3rd molars. If therapy is inadequate, the acute stage may subside and the condition become subacute or chronic. In severe cases there is a fetid odor and a foul taste in the mouth. The treatment of choice is complete elimination of the local irritants by careful and thorough prophylactic procedures. Mild medicaments used locally, as well as antibiotic therapy, may serve as adjuncts to treatment but are of no value if used independently of scaling and polishing. Caustics are contraindicated.

(Center) Gingival specimen from an area of active necrotizing ulcerative gingivitis. It shows the characteristic intercellular coagulation necrosis with the formation of a false membrane containing numerous colonies of organisms. Intense inflammatory response is evident at the base of the ulcer.

(Bottom) Typical picture of chronic necrotizing ulcerative gingivitis that may follow untreated or improperly treated acute cases. The gingival margin, rather than being scalloped, appears as nearly a straight line. This alteration is due to destruction of interproximal and labial marginal gingiva. An attempt at repair may produce pseudopapillae that extend above the interproximal craters, thus obscuring the tissue destruction in these areas.

GINGIVAL ENLARGEMENT

All generalized nonneoplastic increases in gingival bulk are classified as *gingival enlargement,* while focal enlargements are specifically designated. Enlargements due to inflammation may be manifest as hyperemia, hyperplasia, fibrosis, etc. Included among the causes of gingival enlargements are hormonal imbalances of puberty and pregnancy, heredity, administration of phenytoin (Dilantin), cyclosporine or Procardia, and leukemia. Inflammation may be associated with any of these enlargements.

(Top) Pubertal enlargement is associated with altered hormonal balance at puberty. It usually is preceded by some degree of marginal gingivitis. The papillae increase in size, and the gingival margins are thickened as a result of hyperemia and edema. The tissues are soft and bleed readily. Removal of local irritants may produce some improvement, but reestablishment of hormonal balance is essential for complete resolution. This gingival disease is more common in girls than in boys.

(Center) Enlargement of the gingiva associated with pregnancy is similar, clinically and histologically, to pubertal enlargement. It is associated with hormonal activity of pregnancy but, as in pubertal enlargement, usually has local irritating factors contributing to its initiation. Hormonal therapy is not indicated. The disease occurs in about 5% of pregnant women. The enlargement usually subsides after parturition, but local therapy is desirable, along with good oral hygiene, to aid in controlling the associated gingivitis. A few patients with gingival enlargement of pregnancy develop so-called pregnancy tumors (see p. 97).

(Bottom) The most characteristic histologic feature of hormonal gingival enlargement of puberty or pregnancy is the marked vascularity of the tissues, as shown here. The lesion resembles a pyogenic granuloma. The excessive vascularity accounts for the bright red color, and the hyperemia and edema for the enlargement. Obviously, since the enlargement may resolve when the hormones are in normal relation, gingivectomy is not indicated during pregnancy or puberty for this type of enlargement.

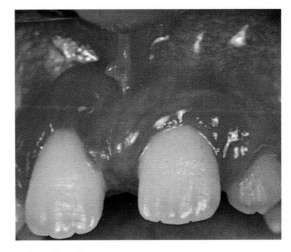

Pubertal Enlargement

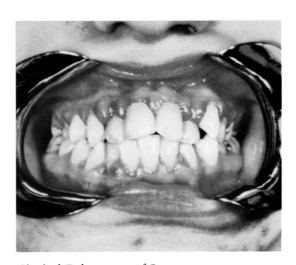

Gingival Enlargement of Pregnancy

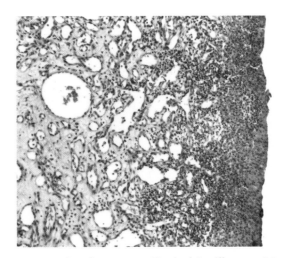

Hormonal Enlargement, Gingival Papilla × 90

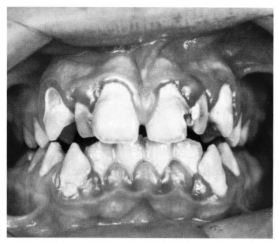

Simple Hyperplastic Gingivitis

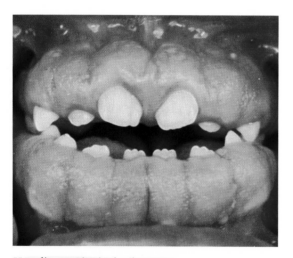

Hereditary Gingival Fibromatosis

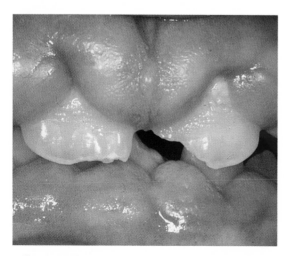

Dilantin Enlargement

GINGIVAL ENLARGEMENT *(continued)*

(Top) Simple hyperplastic gingivitis results from long-continued local irritation. It may be considered a chronic form of simple marginal gingivitis in which the body's response to the continuous irritation is a productive type of inflammation. In simple marginal gingivitis the affected tissue is soft and spongy, the swelling being due to the inflammatory exudate, whereas in simple hyperplastic gingivitis the extensive enlargement of the tissue is firm, being the result of subepithelial fibrosis. In the case illustrated the papillae are markedly increased in size, gingival margins are blunt, and crevices increased in depth. Treatment consists of removal of local irritants, use of periodontal packs, massage, and gingivoplasty.

(Center) In hereditary gingival fibromatosis, usually initiated at the time of eruption of the teeth, the individual has a great genetic propensity for the proliferation of connective tissue in response to minor irritation. Once started, the increase in size of the gingiva is conducive to further local irritation, so that the process becomes progressively more severe. Removal of local irritants may bring improvement, but gingivoplasty is necessary to produce a physiologic contour. Once the excess tissue has been removed, it will be possible to maintain acceptable oral hygiene, which will retard regrowth of tissue.

(Bottom) Phenytoin (Dilantin) enlargement, which closely resembles hereditary gingival fibromatosis both clinically and histologically, occurs in some individuals who are using phenytoin for the control of epilepsy. Other drugs, including cyclosporine, may induce similar enlargements. In this type of gingival disease phenytoin markedly stimulates connective tissue proliferation, resulting in a progressive gingival enlargement that may eventually cover the teeth completely. It is believed that in most instances local irritation is an initiating factor. Plaque control and regular prophylaxis may minimize enlargement and should be initiated as soon as possible after beginning phenytoin therapy. This disease is quite rare in edentulous areas. Gingivoplasty in the presence of continued phenytoin therapy is indicated when there is soft tissue impingement during mastication, but it does not result in a cure.

(Top) In this gingival specimen, from a patient with phenytoin (Dilantin) enlargement, inflammatory cells are seen near the floor of the gingival sulcus (lower left), but the predominant feature is the excessive subepithelial fibrosis. The connective tissue proliferation has caused the gingival tissue to be bulbous and the free margin to be blunt. This photomicrograph could not be distinguished from one of hereditary gingival fibromatosis or possibly from one of simple hyperplastic gingivitis, although in the latter there is often more epithelial hyperplasia, more inflammatory exudate, and less extensive fibrosis.

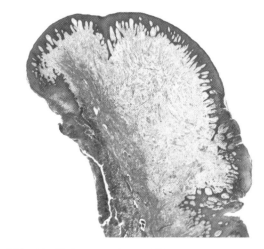

Dilantin Enlargement ×12

(Center) Leukemic enlargement is due to infiltration of the tissues by leukemic cells and usually is associated with severe gingivitis. The gingival color frequently is deep red to purple, and the enlarged tissue may stand away from the teeth, resulting in deep, wide sulci. Edema and hyperemia associated with the gingivitis add to the size of the gingiva. Because of the purpuric tendency (p. 176) there is often severe, spontaneous gingival hemorrhage. Necrosis of the gingiva and adjacent tissues is not uncommon. Early necrosis may be misdiagnosed as necrotizing ulcerative gingivitis. Leukemic enlargement may be seen in any type of leukemia but is most common first in acute monocytic and next myelogenous types. There is no diagnostic characteristic difference in the gingival changes associated with different types of leukemia. Local therapy consists of careful removal of hard and soft deposits and establishing a good oral hygiene. Surgical procedures are contraindicated. The leukemia should be treated by oncologists.

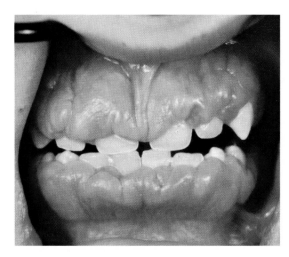

Leukemic Enlargement, Gingiva

(Bottom) Low-power view of gingival specimen (*left*) shows the very heavy infiltration of leukemic cells. The crevicular lining is ulcerated. Under higher magnification (*right*) the atypical leukocytes are seen. The type of cellular infiltration will vary with the type of leukemia (myelogenous, lymphocytic, monocytic), but it is difficult to determine the type of leukemia by examination of a gingival biopsy sample alone. Gingival biopsy is not suggested as a routine diagnostic procedure when leukemia is suspected.

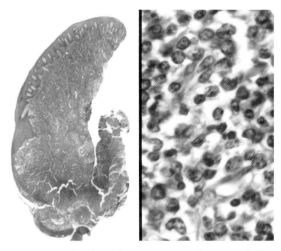

×11　*Leukemic Enlargement, Gingiva*　×560

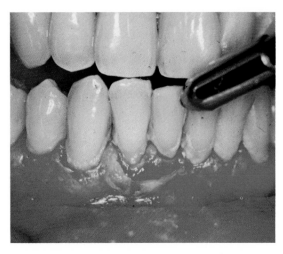

Desquamative Gingivitis

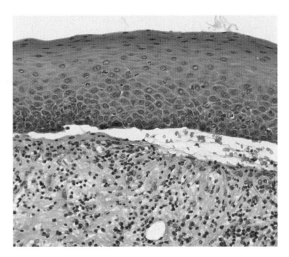

Desquamative Gingivitis, Specimen from Edge of Red Area   ×100

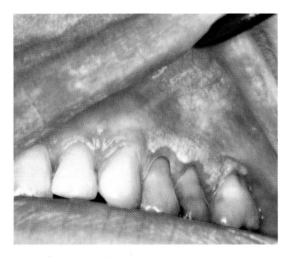

Atrophic Senile Gingivitis

DESQUAMATIVE GINGIVITIS

("GINGIVOSIS")

(Top)   Desquamative gingivitis is characterized by a bullous or vesicular process that causes the epithelium to "desquamate" readily. When the surface is rubbed carefully, a thin vesicle forms and may be ruptured by the very act of rubbing. More vigorous rubbing pulls off the epithelium, leaving a red, shiny, sensitive surface. An airblast introduced into the gingival sulcus usually produces an air-filled bleb. The disease occurs most frequently in middle-aged women; the etiology is unknown, but it may be an immune-related condition. Areas of regeneration and desquamation may give a mottled appearance to the gingiva. Cyclic changes are typical and make evaluation of therapy difficult. In the illustration, several small red denuded areas are apparent. In some cases, at a certain stage of the disease, the entire gingiva may be red and raw from the desquamation. This type of gingival disease should be differentiated from erosive lichen planus of the gingiva.

(Center)   An intense inflammatory infiltrate is present in the connective tissue. The epithelium has separated from the connective tissue. Examination with ultraviolet light would reveal the presence of immunoglobulins at the interface. The histologic findings are similar to those of benign mucous membrane pemphigoid (see p. 123).

ATROPHIC SENILE GINGIVITIS

(Bottom)   Chronic atrophic senile gingivitis is a condition seen in postmenopausal women. It is characterized by atrophy of gingival mucosa, with focal areas of hyperkeratosis. There is usually some gingival recession. In the case pictured the mucosa is thin, shiny, and pale in color. Above the molar and premolar teeth there is a grayish-white rough area of hyperkeratosis. The changes, both clinical and microscopic, are similar to those seen in chronic atrophic senile vaginitis, which is sometimes a concomitant finding. Hormonal therapy, though frequently suggested, is usually of questionable benefit.

(Top)   The dentogingival junction is far down on the cementum, and the surface of the root is covered with calculus and plaque. The epithelium lining the pocket is irregular in pattern, and proliferating projections of this epithelium surround masses of granulation tissue in which there are numerous inflammatory cells. There is a complete loss of arrangement of the periodontal fibers, and much of the alveolar process has been resorbed.

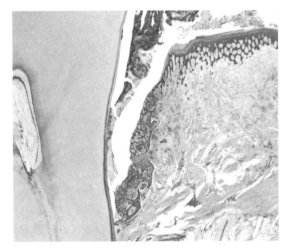

Advanced Periodontitis, Deep Pocket   × 16

(Center)   An infrabony pocket is seen on the left extending below the level of the alveolar crest. The papilla is blunt and folded, and relatively few inflammatory cells are present. The width of the periodontal ligament (on the left) is increased, and there is disorganization of the principal fibers. In the same area the vessels are more numerous and dilated. The interdental septum is markedly resorbed, and fibrosis of some of the marrow spaces is apparent. In this case both vertical and horizontal loss of supporting structures has occurred.

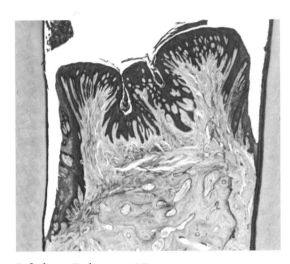

Infrabony Pocket   × 17

(Bottom)   Two teeth with periodontitis in different stages are shown in this photomicrograph. There is marked vertical bone loss next to the tooth at the left with a deep pocket extending far below the alveolar bone crest. The intense inflammation beneath the pocket epithelium makes it difficult to distinguish the epithelial boundary. Connective tissue fiber bundles extend from the alveolar bone crest down along the bone's surface to insert into the cementum below the base of the pocket. Such a pocket is a good candidate for treatment by subgingival curettage. After removal of the pocket epithelium, the residual periodontal ligament participates in organization of the blood clot and regeneration of alveolar bone and fibers. Debris trapped in such narrow, deep pockets may initiate a periodontal abscess. On the left side of the tooth to the right, well oriented periodontal fibers are present on the apical half of the root. Above the alveolar crest there is marked inflammation, but the dentogingival junction has not moved far apically. At the far right a deep pocket is seen, and there is more bone loss. Pocket depth may vary at different places on the same tooth.

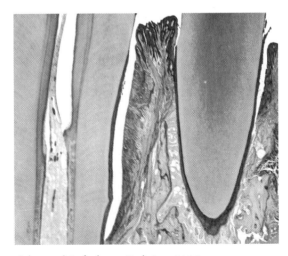

Advanced Infrabony Pocket   × 10

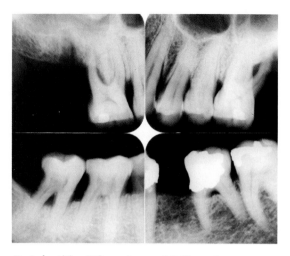

Periodontitis, Bifurcation and Trifurcation Involvement

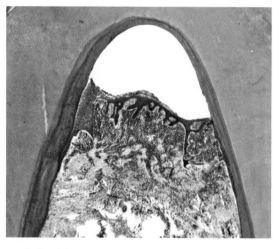

Periodontitis, Horizontal Bone Loss in Bifurcation ×28

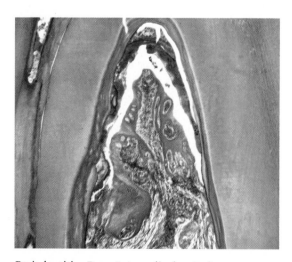

Periodontitis, Deep Interradicular Pockets ×22

PERIODONTAL DISEASE INVOLVING INTERRADICULAR AREAS

When periodontitis has advanced to the degree of involving the interradicular area, treatment and control of the process is difficult. It is important, therefore, to be cognizant of all such areas when analyzing a case and deciding on a plan of treatment. Bifurcation or trifurcation involvement, however, is frequently overlooked, both clinically and radiographically. Inflammatory hyperplasia of gingival tissue may mask the interradicular destruction. In radiographs these areas of decreased density may not be discerned because of improper angulation or the superimposition of radiopaque tissues.

(Top) The upper left film demonstrates that the deep pocket about the distobuccal root extends into the trifurcation. In the lower left radiograph a horizontal type of bone loss is evident, and there is interradicular involvement of both molars—slight in the 1st and advanced in the 2nd. The upper right film illustrates interradicular involvement of the 1st molar and extensive bone loss about the distobuccal root. At the lower right, the molar with the large restoration has a radiolucent area between the roots. This destruction resulted from extension of buccal and lingual pockets.

(Center) Photomicrograph demonstrates advanced horizontal destruction with complete exposure of the bifurcation. The dentogingival junction is comparatively broad on both of the root surfaces. Beneath the irregular covering epithelium is granulation tissue in which there are numerous inflammatory cells. This granulation tissue fills the space formerly occupied by the periodontal ligament and the interradicular bony septum.

(Bottom) This photomicrograph illustrates the histologic appearance of a tooth in which a deep labial or lingual pocket extends into the bifurcation. Calculus, plaque, and soft tissue nearly fill the interradicular area, so that clinically the gingival level might appear normal. If a probe were passed into the crevice, however, the marked destruction would be readily evident. In bifurcation involvement of this configuration, pus is frequently trapped.

TRAUMATISM

Trauma from occlusion exists when abnormal masticatory force has caused injury to the dental pulp, the temporomandibular joint, or the periodontium. It may be a contributing factor and occasionally an initiating factor in periodontal disease. The signs, symptoms, and pathologic changes related to occlusal trauma are due mainly to disturbances in circulation. In the periodontal tissues there may be edema, congestion, hemorrhage, thrombosis, necrosis, atrophy, degeneration, resorption of bone and cementum, and repair.

(Top) Clinical appearance of the gingiva in one stage of traumatism. Excessive orthodontic force had been applied to the tooth. The gingival margins are thick, and some of the interdental papillae are slightly bulbous, although they do not fit the embrasures. Stillman's cleft is apparent in the region of the lower incisors, the one below the lateral incisor being more advanced. These vertical clefts are produced by atrophy of the labial gingiva, together with extension of adjacent hyperplastic tissue over the area of recession. The darker areas on the gingiva are normal melanin pigmentation.

(Center) McCall's festoons (most apparent in this case about the lower anterior teeth) are seen frequently in traumatism but are not pathognomonic of it. These semilunar enlargements of the free gingival margin are the result of compensatory hyperplasia and degeneration of free gingival fibers. Other signs and symptoms of occlusal traumatism are increased mobility of teeth, loss of interproximal contacts, sensitivity of teeth, gingival cyanosis, and disturbances of the temporomandibular joint.

(Bottom) Abnormal force, applied in this case in a distolingual direction, has caused drifting and spacing of the premolars, irregular vertical bone loss, wedge-shaped thickening of the periodontal spaces, and uneven thickness of the lamina dura. If excessive horizontal force is applied in a plane that can be visualized in a radiograph, the typical findings are a cervicolateral wedge-shaped widening of periodontal space on one side and an apicolateral widening on the opposite side.

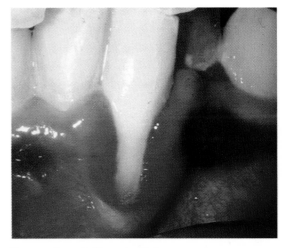

Traumatism, Stillman's Cleft

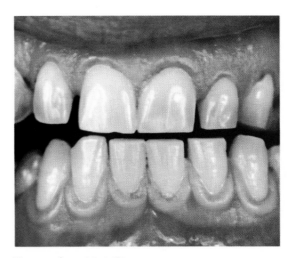

Traumatism, McCall's Festoons

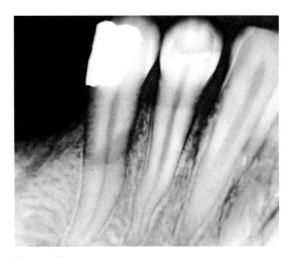

Traumatism

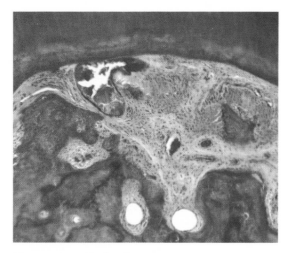

Traumatism, Early Changes ×40

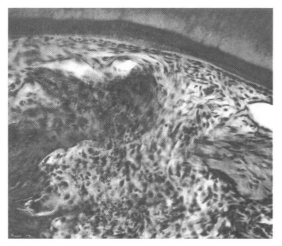

Traumatism, Early Stage of Resolution ×120

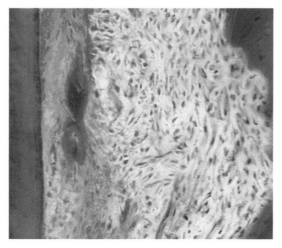

Traumatism, Late Stage of Resolution ×190

TRAUMATISM *(continued)*

A tooth may change position in the jaw without deleterious effect in well-regulated orthodontic treatment, in physiologic mesial drift, and in response to mild alteration of masticatory forces. In these instances there is a slow resorption of the alveolar bone on one side of the tooth and a compensating deposition in response to tension on the opposite side. If a tooth is subjected to severe abnormal stress, however, the periodontal ligament may be compressed markedly, causing impairment of the circulation, which in turn results in degeneration or necrosis. Bone is resorbed extensively in the pressure area and replaced temporarily by granulation tissue. This combination of changes is favorable for the extension of gingival inflammation and may result in deep pocket formation unless the traumatic force and local irritants are eliminated and the tooth stabilized.

(Top) Bifurcation area of a molar tooth showing early changes of traumatism. At extreme left there is hyalin degeneration of the compressed periodontal ligament. Near this area is a large thrombosed vessel (hemorrhage was associated with this vessel in other sections). In most of the photomicrograph the periodontal space is widened due to resorption of the crest of the interradicular septum. In this region young connective tissue and some residual periodontal fibers are present.

(Center) In this case the periodontal ligament and a portion of the bone are replaced by granulation tissue in which there are numerous inflammatory cells. Osteoclastic resorption of the remaining bone is evident. If epithelial rests were present in such an area, they might be stimulated to proliferate.

(Bottom) Healing stage of traumatism from region along the lateral root surface. The alveolar bone has been resorbed beginning on the surfaces next to the periodontal ligament. The fibrous connective tissue replacing the periodontal ligament and extending into the marrow spaces is free of inflammatory cells and shows some degree of maturity. It is loose and, as yet, shows no functional orientation. (Compare normal periodontum, p. 6.)

IV Diseases of the Oral Soft Tissues

INTRODUCTION

This chapter consists of two parts. *Section 1* includes inflammatory, infectious, and reactive lesions of local origin and those that reflect systemic disease. General factors may influence the course and even the initiation of diseases of local origin, and local factors may determine whether any given general disease will show local manifestations and how the lesions progress. Systemic infections that may show local lesions include syphilis, tuberculosis, varicella, measles, and primary herpes.

Section 2 discusses diseases thought to be associated with abnormalities of the immune system—such as scleroderma, pemphigus, and lupus erythematosus—that may have oral signs and symptoms, as well the acquired immune deficiency syndrome (AIDS).

Many disturbances of local origin are due to physical or chemical irritants. Among these are cheek-chewing lesions, hyperplasias from denture irritations, amputation neuromas, and drug burns. Radiation, coal-tar products of tobacco, and electrogalvanism are other local irritants that may be of etiologic importance. Localized infections include actinomycosis, thrush, and, in some instances, sialadenitis. Benign migratory glossitis (geographic tongue) and periadenitis mucosa necrotica recurrens are examples of noninfectious inflammations of local or immune origin.

Not all of the diseases of the oral mucosa and jaws are included in this chapter. Neoplasms, disturbances in development, and diseases relating to the supporting structures of the teeth are discussed elsewhere, and, obviously, many are omitted in a book of limited size.

Diagnosis must be established before definite treatment may be instituted. The diagnosis may be quite obvious, or it may be necessary to carry out definite steps before the disease can be recognized. A detailed history is taken and recorded. The lesion should be examined carefully, both visually and manually, and its characteristics recorded. Radiographic examination is essential when calcified tissues are involved. With the history and the clinical and radiographic examination completed, several possible diagnoses may come to mind, and then it may be necessary to ask additional specific questions or to seek assistance through biopsy or from specific laboratory tests. Even though the diagnosis of a given lesion may appear simple, the capable clinician will seek complete information and think carefully before making a decision.

It is important to be able to recognize the cause of a given oral disease and to distinguish lesions of local origin from those with generalized causes. To do this it is necessary to have a thorough knowledge of those systemic diseases that produce oral lesions and of the appearance of the locally produced disturbances. Obviously, the treatment for diseases of local origin is quite different than that for diseases of systemic origin, although many lesions of systemic origin require local as well as systemic therapy. Failure to recognize the systemic origin of oral ulcers resulting from such diseases as agranulocytosis, syphilis, leukemia, or pernicious anemia may delay initiation of therapy until irreversible changes have occurred. The dentist, as the member of the health services team responsible for the oral cavity, must accept the obligation to diagnose and treat diseases of the oral mucosa and jaw bones and to refer for treatment extraoral diseases with oral manifestations.

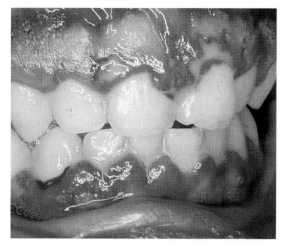

Primary Herpetic Gingivostomatitis

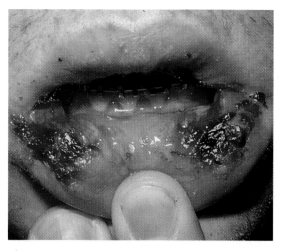

Ruptured, Crusted Herpetic Lesions

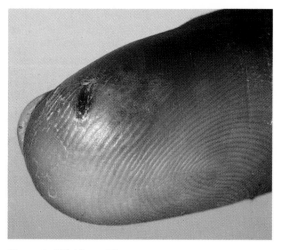

Herpetic Whitlow, Finger

1. INFLAMMATORY, INFECTIOUS, AND REACTIVE CONDITIONS

PRIMARY HERPES SIMPLEX VIRUS (HSV) INFECTION

HSV type 1 produces the most common viral infection in the oral cavity. It most often occurs in children under 6 years of age but can involve older patients. In most children primary infection is subclinical; about 13% of children have had symptomatic herpes by age 9.

(Top) The primary episode is characterized by constitutional symptoms such as malaise, fever and regional lymphadenopathy. Acute ulcerative gingivostomatitis occurs as a result of virus replication in the affected tissues. Vesicular eruptions may occur throughout the mouth.

The gingivae are red and swollen and bleed readily. They may have a mottled appearance, as seen here in the maxillary areas. Touching them or attempting to consume food causes severe pain.

(Center) Vesicles rupture, leaving shallow, painful ulcers. In adolescence and beyond, the primary infection produces an acute tonsillopharyngitis. In most cases the stomatitis resolves within 14 days. Following resolution, antibodies to the virus can be measured. These persist for years. They do not, however, prevent recurrence, as the virus resides in a latent state in the trigeminal ganglion (see p. 87).

(Bottom) Herpetic infection of the digits (herpetic whitlow) occurs through a break in the skin and results from localized virus replication which causes swelling, redness, and tenderness with subsequent vesiculation. Healing follows in 2 weeks; as in other HSV infections, latency and periodic reactivations are common. Herpetic whitlow is a recognized occupational hazard of dental personnel and may be contracted through treatment of patients with oral herpetic lesions. The dentist, hygienist, or assistant in turn, may transmit this infection to other patients.

To prevent this infection, gloves should be used routinely when examining or treating patients.

RECURRENT HERPETIFORM LESIONS

These recurrent oral and labial lesions result from the reactivation of herpes simplex virus residual in the trigeminal ganglion from primary infection (see p. 86). Reactivation of the virus and appearance of the lesions may be associated with upper respiratory infection, tissue manipulation or trauma, fever, exposure to sunlight, gastrointestinal upsets, and menstruation. The recurrent lesions usually are limited in extent, beginning with a slight swelling and a mild burning sensation, followed in a few hours by vesicle formation. In moist areas the thin-walled blisters rupture almost immediately, and on the lips they persist for only a few hours. Unless they become severely infected secondarily, the resultant ulcers remain superficial, healing in 10 to 14 days without scarring. Constitutional symptoms typical of primary herpetic gingivostomatitis are absent in the recurrent disease. Limited clinical trials suggest that antiviral agents decrease the severity of the recurrences and may lengthen the time between recurrent episodes.

(Top) Large vesicle of lip resulting from coalescence of smaller ones. Virus can be isolated from these lesions for several days and can serve as a source of infection for susceptible individuals (newborns and immunosuppressed). In the vesicular stage the lesions of herpes may be dehydrated with absolute alcohol and ether, preventing rupturing and secondary infection. Healing time may be shortened thereby.

(Center) A typical conglomerate lesion of herpes labialis which was initiated by sunlight. Some of the vesicles have already ruptured, fibrin has been deposited, and a crust has been formed.

(Bottom) Recurrent intraoral herpetic lesions tend to develop on oral mucosa that is tightly bound to periosteum. The small vesicles rupture quickly, leaving small red ulcerations.

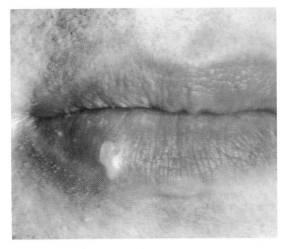

Herpetic Vesicle, Lower Lip

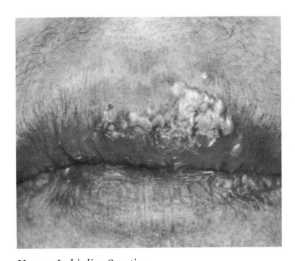

Herpes Labialis, Crusting

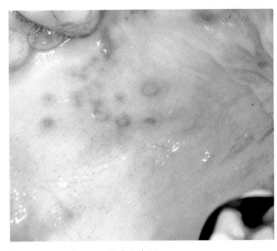

Recurrent Herpes, Palatal Mucosa

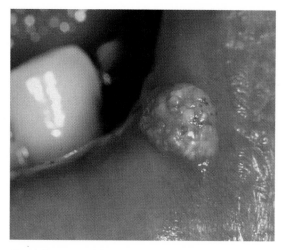

Condyloma acuminatum

VIRAL PAPILLARY LESIONS

(Top) In the oral cavity various epithelial hyperplasias have been associated with human papilloma virus (HPV). Oral condylomas may result from oral–genital contact or from sucking wart-infected fingers. Such lesions are usually exophytic and appear as cauliflower-like processes with narrow stalks. They have a high rate of recurrence. Single oral papillomas, discussed in the chapter on neoplasms (see p. 144), also may demonstrate the presence of HPV antigens, as do certain leukoplakias.

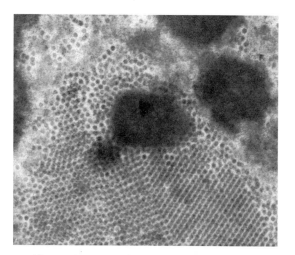

Papilloma virus particles × *74,250*

(Center) Whole virus particles or virus components (particularly viral DNA) have been isolated from oral lesions. More than 50 distinct types of HPV have been identified and associated with specific types of epithelial lesions. HPV-6 or HPV-11 are most commonly believed to be the etiologic agent for condyloma acuminatum.

EXANTHEMS

(Bottom) These infectious diseases with accompanying skin lesions occur primarily in children but may appear later in persons who escape the diseases during childhood. In chickenpox (varicella) the cutaneous eruption frequently is associated with coalescing vesicular oral lesions, as seen here in the palate. In measles (rubeola) small bluish-white spots on bright red bases (Koplik spots) may be seen, usually adjacent to Stensen's duct, during the late prodromal and early eruptive stage. Small petechial spots at the junction of the hard and soft palate may be seen in German measles (rubella).

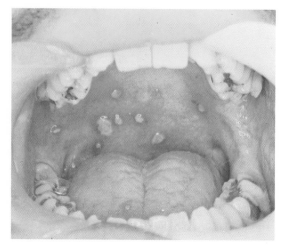

Chickenpox, (Varicella), Palate

ACTINOMYCOSIS

Actinomycosis, a deep microbial infection caused by the anaerobic *Actinomyces israeli (A. bovis),* is characterized by granulomatous lesions that eventually suppurate. Abdominal, thoracic, and cervicofacial forms of the disease occur; the last is by far the most common. In cervicofacial actinomycosis there is often a history of tooth extraction, and it is believed that *Actinomyces,* which are common inhabitants of the oral cavity, may gain access to bone through the extraction wound. One or more months later the infection becomes manifest by the appearance of a slowly progressive, very firm swelling of the cheek or neck. Pus is evacuated externally from several sinuses when the lesion softens.

(Top) The cervicofacial swelling is of a typical light-purplish color, and at its superior and inferior aspects draining sinuses are apparent. The pus in this disease is scant but very thick. It contains tiny yellow granules (colonies of *A. israeli*) that may be seen grossly and resemble sulfur granules. Contiguous tissue gradually becomes involved, and more sinuses form. Cervicofacial actinomycosis has a good prognosis but often runs a protracted course.

(Center) Enlargement of a "sulfur granule" in a tissue section. The granule is surrounded by pus, at the periphery of which are numerous lipid-containing macrophages. One should suspect actinomycosis when examining granulation tissue that has numerous microabscesses and abundant foam cells, but the diagnosis should not be made unless the causative organisms are found. The granule is composed of numerous gram-positive, branching, filamentous organisms. At the edge of the granule the peripheral ends of the organisms may protrude slightly as eosinophilic, club-shaped enlargements.

CANDIDIASIS

(Bottom) Candidiasis (candidosis, thrush, moniliasis) on the tongue of a young child. The white covering resembles a mat of milk curds and, as seen in this picture, leaves a red raw surface when scraped off. *Candida albicans,* a normal inhabitant of the mouth, is the cause. It produces disease in immunosuppressed patients (including those with AIDS), and when long treatment with antibiotics has eliminated most of the competitive oral flora. *Candida* often are involved in denture sore mouth. The commissural area is frequently involved.

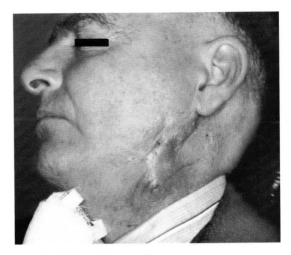

Cervicofacial Actinomycosis

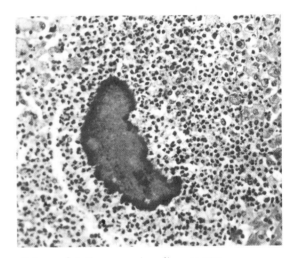

Colony of Actinomyces israeli   ×220

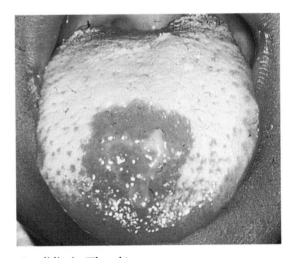

Candidiasis (Thrush)

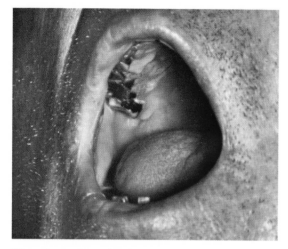

Histoplasmosis, Palatal Mucosa

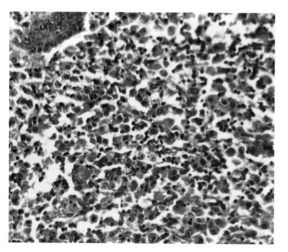

Histoplasmosis, Biopsy Specimen from Oral Lesion   ×215

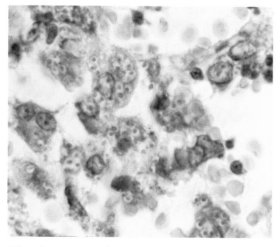

Histoplasma Capsulatum, Giemsa's Stain   ×970

HISTOPLASMOSIS

Histoplasmosis, a specific infectious disease that affects mainly the reticuloendothelial system, is caused by the fungus *Histoplasma capsulatum*. At the site of entry (often the oral cavity) a slowly enlarging, indolent ulcer usually develops. The causative organisms may become widely disseminated, involving in particular the lungs, liver, spleen, and bone marrow. As the disease progresses there is anemia, leukopenia, enlargement of liver and spleen, low-grade fever, and continuing weight loss. This classic, disseminated form of the disease may run a fatal course. If the disease remains localized, the prognosis is good. In certain areas of the United States nearly half of the adults give a positive reaction to the histoplasmin skin test. If a positive skin test actually is indicative of a previous infection, then a very mild, asymptomatic form of the disease is quite common. Dermal sensitivity apparently develops slowly, for individuals with the active disease frequently are negative reactors.

(Top)   In this case of disseminated histoplasmosis, ulceration of the gingiva and palatal mucosa was the primary manifestation of the disease. The lesion was first noticed 2 mo previously and had increased gradually in size. This patient's liver and spleen slowly enlarged, and there was radiographic evidence of lung involvement. The patient died of the disease 6 mo after the appearance of the oral lesion.

(Center)   Infection by *Histoplasma capsulatum* results in the formation of a granulomatous lesion characterized by moderate vascularity, epithelioid cells, caseation necrosis, and numerous macrophages containing the fungus. In the photomicrograph many large macrophages are apparent, but at this magnification the fungus cannot be visualized.

(Bottom)   At higher magnification the organisms (round bodies 1 to 5 μ in diameter) can be seen packed in the macrophages. Each has a centrally placed nucleus and a clear, thick capsule. The organisms may easily be overlooked in routine hematoxylin and eosin preparations, especially if they are scarce.

TUBERCULOSIS

(Top) Bilateral cervical tuberculous lymphadenitis in a young boy. This form of the disease is due to infection with the bovine strain of tubercle bacilli, usually as a result of drinking milk from tuberculous cows. The microorganisms enter the body through the tonsillar tissue constituting Waldeyer's ring, and some of them reach the regional lymph nodes and produce secondary lesions. The involved nodes gradually enlarge; they are hard and discrete at first but later fuse, become soft (due to caseation necrosis), and finally rupture to the surface.

(Center) Tuberculous ulcer with a typical ragged, undermined border. This type of ulcer usually has a gelatinous base and is painful. Occasionally an oral tuberculous lesion is papular in structure. Oral lesions in this disease usually are associated with pulmonary tuberculosis and result from hematogenous spread of the infection or from inoculation of small abrasions by infected sputum. Lesions may occur anywhere in the oral cavity; they are rare, but if present, they frequently involve the tongue. They may occur as periapical lesions.

Tubercle bacilli (human or bovine strains) may enter the body by way of the respiratory tract, the alimentary tract, or the skin. Infection of the lung by the human type of bacillus is by far the most frequent form of this disease in humans. Many individuals have a tuberculous infection of the lung in early childhood. The primary focus is usually located in the midportion of the lung just beneath the pleura. Regional lymph nodes also become involved. The tuberculous nodes and the lung focus constitute the primary or juvenile complex. On recovery the person usually has some degree of immunity to the tubercle bacillus, though in some cases a hypersensitivity is developed. Reinfection may occur in adult life.

(Bottom) Photomicrograph showing epithelioid cells, lymphocytes, and a typical Langhans' giant cell with nuclei arranged peripherally with a horseshoe appearance. In the inset, acid-fast tubercle bacilli (red) are demonstrated in tissue stained by the Ziehl-Neelsen method.

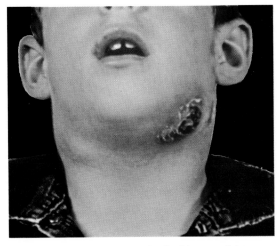

Cervical Tuberculous Lymphadenitis (Scrofula)

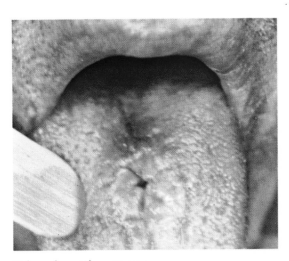

Tuberculous Ulcer, Tongue

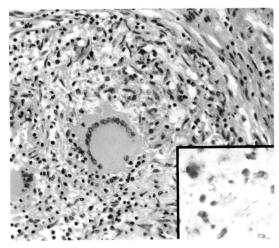

Langhans' Giant Cell ×300
Tubercle Bacilli ×1000

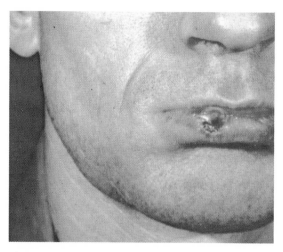

Chancre, Lip

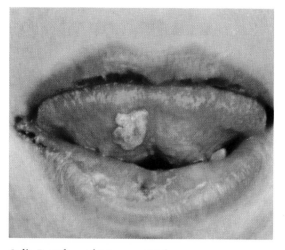

Split Papule and Mucous Patch

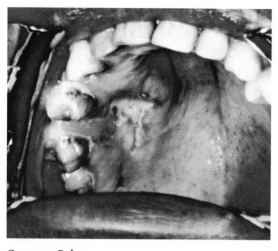

Gumma, Palate

SYPHILIS

(Top) This venereal disease caused by *Treponema pallidum* has three stages. *The primary lesion*, or chancre, appears at the site of invasion 2 to 6 wk after inoculation. The chancre is raised and hard and usually measures less than 1/2 in in diameter. After 2 or 3 days it ulcerates and is covered by a glazed crust. The base is very firm and, when palpated, feels like a rubber button under the tissue. Within a few days after the appearance of the primary lesion one or more regional lymph nodes enlarge (satellite bubo). The chancre will disappear, even without treatment, in 2 to 5 wk, and the patient may not have a positive serology until this time. The lips and fingers are the most frequent sites of extragenital chancres. Clinically, a lip chancre, as shown in the picture, is difficult to differentiate from carcinoma (see p. 168) and from a secondarily infected herpetic lesion. The diagnosis of an oral lesion as syphilis on the basis of dark-field examination alone should be made with great caution, because of the morphologic similarity between *T. pallidum* and oral spirochetes.

(Center) Following the disappearance of the primary lesion there is a period of from 2 mo to 1 yr in which there are no clinical manifestations of the disease. The *secondary stage* often begins with symptoms similar to those of an attack of influenza—sore throat, neuralgic pains, and headache. These are followed by a generalized lymphadenopathy and a mucocutaneous eruption. In the picture two types of secondary oral lesions are demonstrated. A split papule is seen at the corner of the mouth, half being on each lip. A mucous patch is apparent on the underside of the tongue. The latter lesion, which is usually slightly raised, begins as a macule, papule, or vesicle; it rapidly ulcerates and becomes covered with a grayish-white membrane. It is highly infectious.

(Bottom) The gumma, a localized lesion of *tertiary syphilis,* is so named because it has the consistency of firm rubber. This lesion, is especially destructive to bone and cartilage. Gumma of the palate may perforate the bone; involvement of the vomer may result in a collapse of the bridge of the nose ("saddle nose"). Histologically, the gumma is somewhat similar to the lesions of tuberculosis. The primary and secondary lesions of syphilis are characterized by a marked vascularity and a preponderance of plasma cells, which are usually in perivascular arrangement.

CHEEK AND TONGUE CHEWING

(Top) Three weeks before this picture was taken the patient severely lacerated his tongue while chewing. The area of injury became secondarily infected, and this large ulcerated lesion with a raised, rolled border developed. The surrounding tissue was firm to palpation. Such a lesion cannot be differentiated clinically from carcinoma (see p. 169) and should be considered malignant until proven otherwise by histologic examination. This lesion healed following penicillin therapy, but that treatment was not instituted until it had been established that the lesion was inflammatory and not neoplastic. In cases such as this, in which there is a strong clinical impression of malignancy, it is good practice to perform a biopsy.

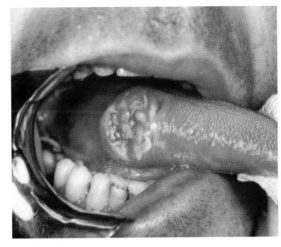

Traumatic Ulcer, Tongue

(Center) Some people have a habit of nibbling unconsciously on the cheek mucosa. As demonstrated in the illustration, this may produce a thin, rough keratotic film in the area irritated. Fragments of epithelium, attached at one end, are often seen in these cases due to continual nibbling on the same area. Grasping these shreds of tissue with the teeth and stripping them off leaves red, raw, eroded areas. Patients usually deny the nibbling habit, but the lesions resulting from it are generally very characteristic. Chewing of the cheek may result in an enlargment.

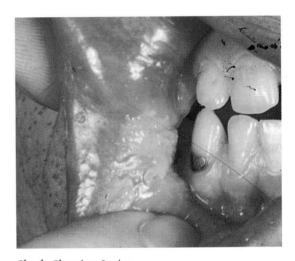

Cheek Chewing Lesion

(Bottom) A large ulcerated lesion that resulted from a single act of trauma. Most people at some time or other bite the cheek inadvertently while chewing. Lesions produced by these injuries are usually not severe, and they heal rapidly. In the case illustrated, however, the teeth probably penetrated deep into the tissue, causing vascular damage. The thrombosis that followed deprived the area of its nutrient supply, and necrosis resulted. This type of lesion tends to be expansile for a few days after the injury. Due to secondary infection and the extensiveness of these lesions, they usually heal slowly, with the production of abundant granulation tissue. Because of their persistence and their indurated borders, they may simulate carcinoma clinically.

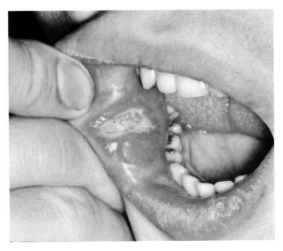

Traumatic Ulcer, Cheek

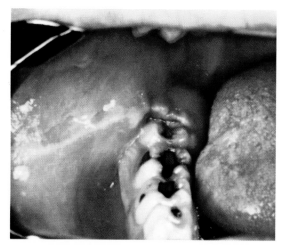

Linea Alba

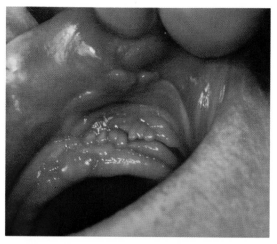

Inflammatory Hyperplasia, Alveolar Mucosa

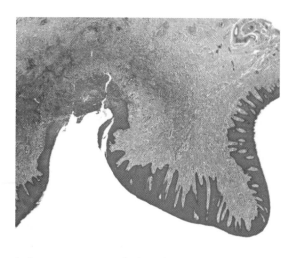

Inflammatory Hyperplasia, Alveolar Mucosa   × 13

CHEEK AND TONGUE CHEWING
(continued)

(Top)   The soft, linear streak of parakeratin seen in the buccal mucosa at the occlusal line is frequently termed the linea alba. These lesions usually occur in individuals with thick cheeks that are closely adapted to the buccal surfaces of the teeth. The line may be initiated by irritation from sharp buccal cusps. This condition may be intensified by the habit of sucking and chewing on the cheeks.

HYPERPLASIA FROM DENTURE IRRITATION

(Center)   The numerous curtainlike folds of excess tissue are the result of wearing an ill-fitting maxillary denture. Originally there may be a small ulcer (denture cut), but as the soft tissue continues to be irritated by the denture flange, a productive inflammation results. This type of hyperplasia may be seen about the anterior part of a complete maxillary denture when the patient has natural anterior mandibular teeth but no posterior replacements. Inflammatory hyperplasia of this sort, while basically similar to that occurring elsewhere in response to chronic irritation, has been termed *epulis fissuratum* because of the cleft or clefts found in the enlargement.

(Bottom)   A fissure that accommodated the edge of a denture is apparent along the lower border of this cross-sectioned biopsy specimen. At the deepest part of the crevice there is ulceration. The whole specimen is heavily infiltrated with inflammatory cells. The bulbous enlargement at the right would be seen clinically as a fold of tissue hanging over the periphery of the denture. The covering epithelium is slightly hyperplastic, but this soft tissue enlargement is mainly the result of fibrous tissue proliferation and inflammation.

(Top) Inflammatory papillary hyperplasia of the palatal mucosa frequently is observed under ill-fitting dentures, especially those having a relief chamber. The hyperplasia is produced in response to irritation from movement of the denture and from accumulating debris. *Candida albicans* may contribute to the inflammation. The polypoid masses usually are intensely red, soft, and freely movable. If the denture is not worn for several days, the inflammation will subside, and the size of the papillomatous nodules may be reduced. They seldom disappear completely and should be removed surgically.

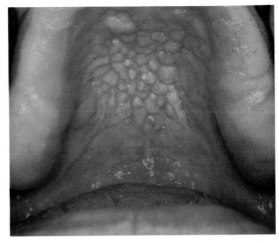

Inflammatory Papillary Hyperplasia, Palate

(Center) This is a photomicrograph of a section of tissue removed from the palate in the above case. The surface epithelium along the lower border of the specimen is hyperplastic, and long, slender rete pegs extend into the lamina propria, which is quite vascular and very heavily infiltrated with inflammatory cells. It is apparent that there has been a proliferation of connective tissue which has contributed to the formation of the papillomatous masses. Some of these may show pseudoepitheliomatous hyperplasia in the epithelium, but frank carcinoma is rare. Note the colonies of organisms along the surface of the lesion.

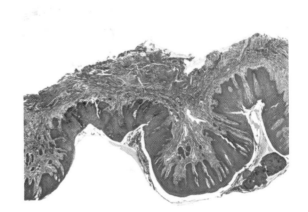

Inflammatory Papillary Hyperplasia   × 17

SELF-INFLICTED TRAUMA DURING ANESTHESIA

(Bottom) This lesion resulted from biting the lip while it was anesthetized. Such a penetrating wound with superficial secondary infection is occasionally found in children following their first experience with mandibular block anesthesia. The child may bite the anesthetized lip inadvertently while eating or, fascinated with the tingling sensation, may playfully chew on it much harder than realized because no pain is felt. In most instances, patient and parents are unaware that the wound was self-inflicted and may believe that some accident occurred during dental treatment. Emphatically forewarning both the child and the parents of the injury that can be produced by biting the lip will often prevent its occurrence.

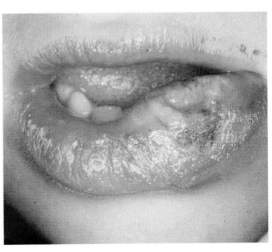

Self-Inflicted Trauma During Anesthesia

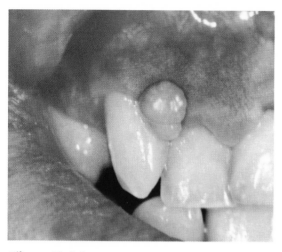

Fibrous Nodule

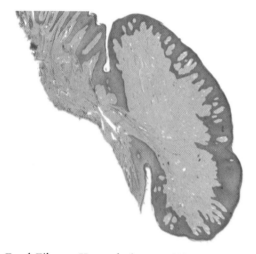

Focal Fibrous Hyperplasia   × 17

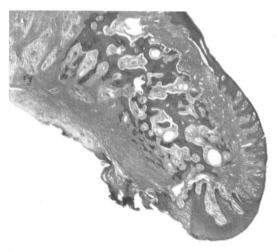

Peripheral Ossifying Fibroma   × 20

FOCAL FIBROUS HYPERPLASIA

(FIBROUS NODULE)

The lesion is due to a low-grade irritation of long duration that results in an exuberant overgrowth of granulation tissue with fibrous organization. It is similar to the fibrotic nodules produced by cheek chewing (see p. 93). It is not a true neoplasm but is an exaggeration of the repair process. Surgical removal usually is indicated. Formerly, any benign gingival enlargement was termed *epulis.*

(Top)   A slightly lobulated fibrous nodule located between the maxillary right canine and the lateral incisor. It is firm, pedunculated, and light pink in color. The surface of these lesions may become ulcerated because of trauma. They may slowly increase in size if the irritating factor (usually in the gingival sulcus) is still present.

(Center)   This photomicrograph is a low-power view of the nodule seen in the top picture. At the upper left is a portion of the alveolar mucosa, and at the other end of the cut surface is part of the interdental papilla. The oval nodule arising from the gingiva is composed of dense fibrous connective tissue. This particular lesion is of long duration and static. In other instances histologic examination might reveal more epithelial hyperplasia and young proliferating connective tissue heavily infiltrated with inflammatory cells. A fibrous nodule is sometimes referred to as a gingival fibroma, but in no sense is it a true neoplasm. It is not necessary to sacrifice teeth in the removal of this lesion, for it has a superficial origin. It may recur, however, unless the base is completely excised and the source of irritation eliminated.

(Bottom)   In the central portion of another gingival enlargement clinically similar to that seen in the top picture, an extensive amount of trabecular bone is evident. Ossification occurred because young connective tissue cells differentiated into osteoblasts. In addition to ectopic bone formation, mucoid degeneration and dystrophic calcification are relatively frequent findings in reactive growths. This one might be termed *peripheral ossifying fibroma* although it is not a neoplasm.

PYOGENIC GRANULOMA

("PREGNANCY TUMOR")

(Top) This entity, which occurs in both skin and mucous membrane, may be sessile or pedunculated. It may vary in diameter from a few millimeters to 2 or 3 cm. The lesion is usually ulcerated but is sometimes covered by a very thin layer of epithelium. It may be red, purple, or brown in color and have a smooth, granular, or lobulated surface. These lesions tend to bleed easily when manipulated and will recur quickly if not adequately removed. Histologic examination of the lesion reveals an outgrowth of granulomatous tissue characterized by extreme endothelial proliferation. At the edge of the lesion the epithelium often tends to proliferate inward as if to separate the granulomatous mass from the underlying normal tissue. Near the surface of the overgrowth the connective tissue is young and delicate and there are numerous small vascular spaces. If the lesion is ulcerated, there are many neutrophils in this area. In some regions there may be masses of endothelial cells not organized into vascular structures. Near the base of the lesion the vascular spaces are large and thin-walled and are surrounded by mature connective tissue stroma.

(Center) Topographic view of a pyogenic granuloma. It is covered by very thin epithelium, and the marked vascularity of the lesion is readily apparent. Pyogenic granuloma and granuloma gravidarum (pregnancy tumor) are identical histologically. In pregnant patients excision should be delayed, if possible, until after parturition, at which time the lesion usually undergoes partial involution.

(Bottom) Higher magnification of the central portion of the above lesion. In the granulation tissue are a few lymphocytes and neutrophils, but most of the large cells are of the endothelial type. Some of these are forming very small vascular channels but most are not so organized.

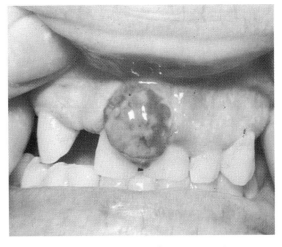

Pyogenic Granuloma (Granuloma Pyogenicum), Gingiva

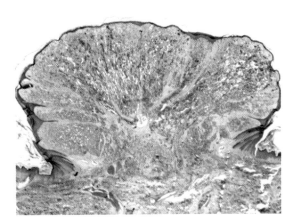

Pyogenic Granuloma × 10

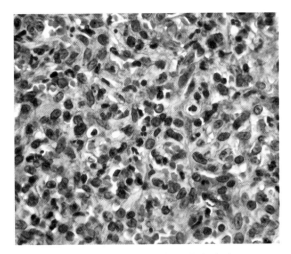

Pyogenic Granuloma, Marked Endothelial Proliferation × 450

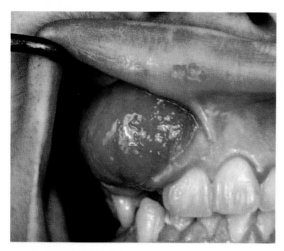

Giant Cell Granuloma

GIANT CELL GRANULOMA

(Top) Peripheral giant cell granuloma is a non-neoplastic enlargement characterized by proliferating fibroblasts that form a stroma containing numerous multinucleated giant cells. Clinically, the lesion usually is soft, sessile, or slightly pedunculated and purple to deep-red in color. It is often fairly large and is relatively common in women and children. It may become ulcerated and bleed readily. This entity may involve the periodontal ligament but also occurs in edentulous areas. Occasionally it may cause superficial bone destruction. It recurs rapidly if not completely removed. Sometimes the lesions stop growing, fibrose, and become indistinguishable from fibrous nodules.

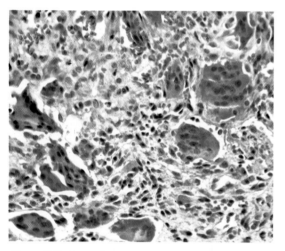

Giant Cell Granuloma ×230

(Center) This photomicrograph demonstrates the spindle cell stroma and the multinucleated giant cells that are typical of this lesion. Other characteristic features of this entity are hemosiderin-filled macrophages and numerous red blood cells located in sinusoidal spaces and extravascularly. Whether the giant cells are osteoclasts or of the foreign body type is in dispute. A histologically similar lesion in the jaws, designated as a central giant cell granuloma, is indistinguishable from a "brown tumor" occurring in hyperparathyroidism (see p. 136).

DIFFERENTIAL DIAGNOSIS

(Bottom) Several of the entities discussed on pages 96, 97, and 98 can present very similar clinical appearances. In the case illustrated, a pyogenic granuloma, a peripheral ossifying fibroma, a traumatized fibrous nodule, and a peripheral giant granuloma should all be considered. Biopsy, which is essential for definitive diagnosis, revealed this lesion to be a peripheral giant cell granuloma. The blue color is frequently seen in this growth but is not pathognomic.

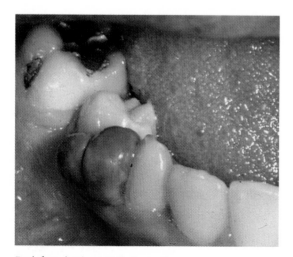

Peripheral Giant Cell Granuloma

MUCOUS EXTRAVASATION PHENOMENON

(MUCOCELE)

(Top)   Spherical swelling of the lower lip due to an abnormal collection of mucin in the underlying tissues. This enlargement might be confused clinically with a mixed tumor of salivary gland origin (see p. 161) or with a lipoma (see p. 146). A mixed tumor, however, is quite firm to palpation. A lipoma is soft and may be yellow, whereas a mucocele is fluctuant and often has a slight bluish tinge. Oral mucoceles occur most frequently in the lower lip but may be found wherever there is salivary gland tissue. Trauma is the most likely cause of mucoceles. Mucin escapes into the tissues surrounding the gland, coagulates, causes an inflammatory reaction, and is walled off by granulation tissue. Obstructing the duct in laboratory animals failed to produce similar lesions, and the results of experimentally severing salivary gland ducts in laboratory animals have been variable.

(Center)   Topographic view of a superficially located mucocele. The surface epithelium (purple-staining border near top of picture) is very thin over the summit of the enlargement. The greater part of the specimen consists of a mass of light bluish-pink-staining homogeneous material (mucin) confined by a capsule of fibrous connective tissue. Inferior to the mucocele are striated muscle fibers (red) and salivary gland tissue (blue). An epithelial lining may be present in small mucoceles but is seldom seen in large ones. Clinically, the lesion shown here would probably appear blue because it is located near the surface, but one more deeply situated would not exhibit that feature. Mucoceles of long duration sometimes become organized and then are represented by a fibrotic nodule.

(Bottom)   A large mucous retention cyst located in the floor of the mouth is generally termed a *ranula* because of its supposed resemblance to the ventral surface of a frog. Ranulas are usually associated with the sublingual glands and may be unilateral, like the one pictured, or they may involve the whole floor of the mouth. When superficial they appear as blue or purplish-red enlargements. Occasionally they are congenital.

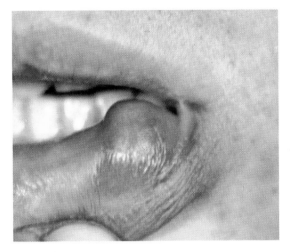

Mucocele, Lip

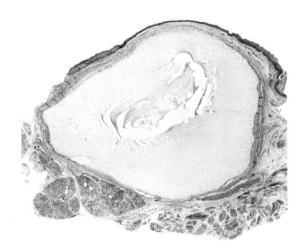

Mucocele   × 9

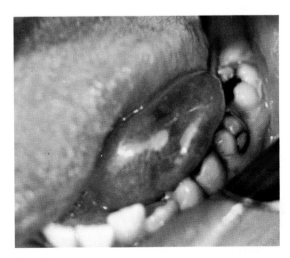

Ranula

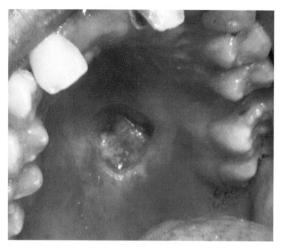

Necrotizing Sialometaplasia, Palate

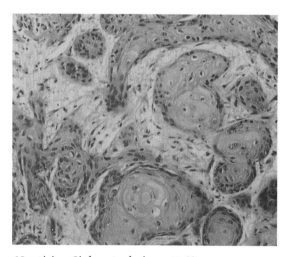

Necotizing Sialometaplasia   × 40

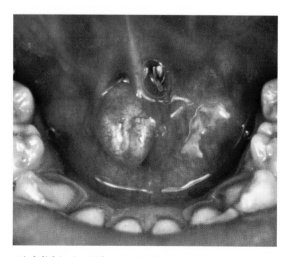

Sialolithiasis, Wharton's Duct

NECROTIZING SIALOMETAPLASIA

(Top) Necrotizing sialometaplasia is a benign inflammatory disease of the glands of the palate, characterized clinically by a raised tumorlike mass, frequently with a deep surface ulcer. Since the ulcerations are persistent, a clinical diagnosis of malignancy is commonly tendered. In the case pictured here, the ulcerated growth had been present for over 2 wk.

(Center) Two processes produce the characteristic histopathologic pattern of necrotizing sialometaplasia. First there is necrosis (tissue death) of lobules of accessory salivary glands in the palate. Second there is a squamous epithelial cell proliferation replacing some acini as they become depleted of their original cells. In addition there is an inflammatory cell component that infiltrates the area, along with granulation tissue. The cause is not known, but it is thought that some factor or factors interrupt the vascular supply to a particular area, leading to necrosis, inflammation, and attempts at tissue repair, which include metaplastic changes in salivary ducts. Because there is mucus pooling following the necrosis of the secretory elements, and squamous metaplasia of remaining ductal elements, some cases have been erroneously diagnosed as mucoepidermoid carcinoma or squamous cell carcinoma. A correct diagnosis is necessary to prevent the possibility of inappropriate therapy. The ulcer heals slowly (about 6 to 8 weeks).

SIALOLITHIASIS

Stones may form in any of the major or minor salivary glands or their excretory ducts. The submandibular gland and Wharton's duct are by far the most frequently involved. The most common manifestation of ductal calculi, which do not generally cause a complete obstruction, is enlargement of the gland during eating. The glandular swelling diminishes between meals as the entrapped saliva is gradually excreted. When such swelling occurs, there may be severe pain. Histologic examination of a decalcified stone reveals that calcified material has been deposited in circular layers.

(Bottom) A relatively large salivary stone is apparent in Wharton's duct. The overlying tissue is distended, and capillaries are quite evident. Removal can be accomplished readily by stabilizing the stone and incising down to it. The wound should not be sutured, for obstruction of the duct is apt to result. Small stones in this location may sometimes be milked out of the duct.

(Top) Occlusal radiograph revealing ovoid, opaque areas which are salivary calculi in the submandibular duct. When salivary stones are suspected, care should be taken in the angulation of the x-ray tube so that the mandible is not superimposed over the area in question. It is believed that salivary stones develop as a result of deposition of mineral salts on a nidus of organic material.

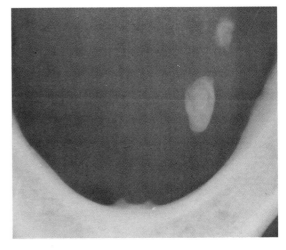

Salivary Calculi

TRAUMATIC (AMPUTATION) NEUROMA

This entity is not a neoplasm, as the name might imply, but an exaggerated response to nerve injury. Peripheral nerves have a great propensity for regeneration. When such a nerve is severed, both parts degenerate—the peripheral end completely, and the proximal portion back to the first node of Ranvier. After degeneration is completed, the stump of the nerve begins to grow along its old course and, if not impeded, will completely reinnervate the part. If the regenerating nerve tissue meets some obstruction such as dense scar tissue, it may continue to proliferate locally, and a nodule of nerve and scar tissue may be formed. The mass thus produced is a traumatic neuroma. If sensory nerves are involved, pain is felt upon pressure. Traumatic neuromas frequently occur in amputation stumps. The most common oral site is over the mental foramen in edentulous mouths, but they may occur wherever a tooth has been removed.

(Center) A tangled mass of nerve and scar tissue forming an ovoid enlargement at the end of a nerve. This appeared as a slowly enlarging, painful nodule in the neck following by 2 yr the dissection of cervical lymph nodes in the treatment of carcinoma, metastatic from the tongue.

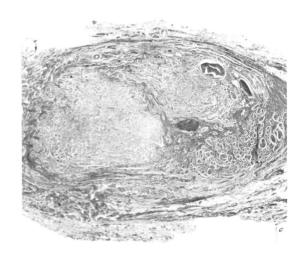

Traumatic Neuroma × 12

(Bottom) Photomicrograph of a portion of the above traumatic neuroma showing intermingling nerve elements and scar tissue. The reddish-purple areas are dense fibrous connective tissue; the light-lavender-staining components are nerve fascicles. With the stain used, the axon cylinders are not apparent at this magnification. The small, dark-staining, wavy, spindle-shaped structures are Schwann cell nuclei.

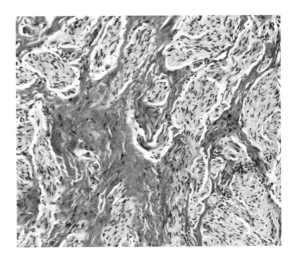

Traumatic Neuroma, Higher Magnification of Same Specimen × 100

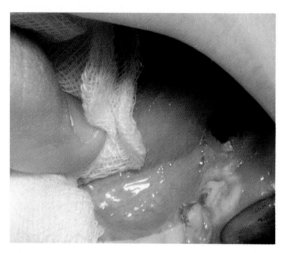

Thermal Burn, Methyl Methacrylate

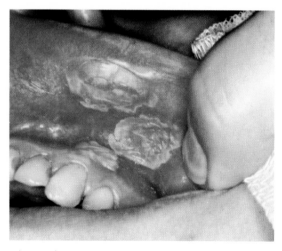

Chemical Burn, Aspirin

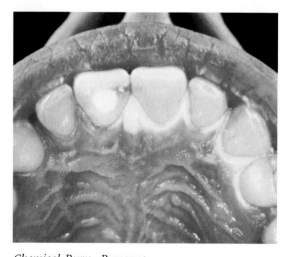

Chemical Burn, Pyrozone

THERMAL BURNS

(Top) Extensive thermal burns do not occur often in the oral cavity, principally because of its inaccessibility to most of the severe thermal hazards. Minor burns, as from very hot beverages or foods, occasionally occur on the palatal or labial mucosa even though this tissue is somewhat protected from thermal injury by its moist surface. Severe sloughing of the oral mucosa from flash burns occasionally is seen in combat personnel. Burns of varying degrees of severity may result from careless application of cautery, using dental instruments that are too hot, dropping hot wax on the tissues, or using impression material that is at too high a temperature. In the patient shown, the coagulation of the gingival mucosa resulted from attempting to fabricate a temporary bridge using methyl methacrylate. Within 24 hr all of the coagulated material sloughed, exposing the underlying bone.

CHEMICAL BURNS

(Center) The placing of an aspirin tablet in the mucobuccal fold to alleviate dental pain is a common but unwarranted practice. It usually causes coagulation of cytoplasm, producing a discrete white area corresponding roughly to the size and shape of the tablet. The lesions generally are superficial unless the aspirin tablets are used repeatedly in this improper manner. If powdered aspirin is applied, a larger area of the mucosa will be involved. Chemical burns may also be produced by many other substances; the most frequently encountered are caused by sodium perborate, phenol, toothache drops, and zinc chloride. The lesions are not specific for each drug, and it is necessary to question the patient to determine the causative agent.

(Bottom) This chemical burn was produced by Pyrozone, which was being used for bleaching the pulpless maxillary right central incisor. The coagulated tissue is apparent along the gingival margins of all the upper left anterior teeth. The pattern of the affected area corresponds to the typical distribution of a liquid escaping through an improperly adapted rubber dam. Currently, hydrogen peroxide 30% (Superoxol) is used for bleaching teeth, but it, too, may cause a tissue burn if used carelessly.

PIGMENTATION FROM HEAVY METALS(INCLUDING DENTAL MATERIALS)

Heavy metals may localize in the oral mucosa as circulating metallic salts attracted to areas of inflammation (anachoresis), or may be introduced directly from dental or surgical procedures. Bismuth and silver salts used therapeutically and ingested or inhaled lead may localize in the gingiva, producing a blue or gray line. Bismuth is an ingredient of some agents used to treat gastric disturbances.

(Top) More commonly, heavy metals are introduced directly into the oral soft tissues from silver amalgam or other dental materials, producing a permanent discoloration (tattoo). Alloys to which porcelain is fused may contain chrome, cobalt, or nickel. Gold particles can be introduced. Some dental cements contain zinc; endodontic preparations may contain zinc or arsenic. Since these materials are placed in the subepithelial connective tissue the pigment is permanent unless removed surgically. The gingival pigmentation in this photograph was due to the accidental introduction of amalgam during periodontal surgery.

(Center) The pigmentation is produced by the formation of insoluble silver salts, which are deposited on the collagen fibers of the lamina propria. There is little or no tissue reaction to this foreign material. Silver salts ingested for therapeutic purposes may accumulate in the subepithelial connective tissue, giving a bronze appearance to the skin. This generalized bronze pigmentation is permanent. The condition is called argyria or argyrosis.

(Bottom) Localized tattoos are frequently seen in edentulous areas, probably resulting from the accidental incorporation of amalgam into tissues during extraction (*left*). A dental radiograph of the area may reveal the presence of amalgam particles (*right*). These pigmented areas need not be removed unless there are cosmetic reasons or the particles of amalgam interfere with the seating of a prosthetic appliance.

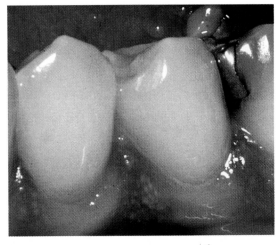

Amalgam Pigmentation　macule

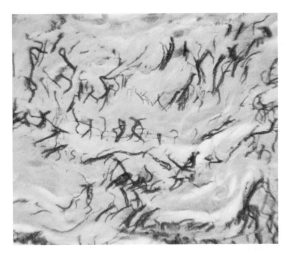

Localized Argyrosis　×100

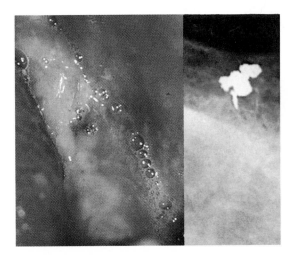

Amalgam in Tissues (left) and in Radiograph (right)

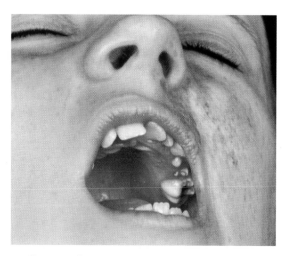

Radiation Effect—Left Side of Face and Maxilla

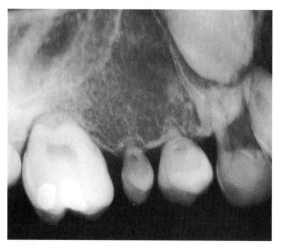

Malformed Teeth, Effect of Radiation

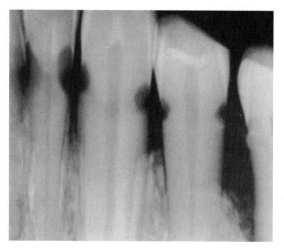

Cervical Destruction Resulting from Extensive Radiation

RADIATION EFFECT

Experimental studies and clinical evidence indicate that radiant energy may interfere with normal development of the teeth. Clinically, this energy usually is derived from a source being used in treatment of neoplastic disease. The effect of radiation on developing teeth depends on the dosage given, the stage of tooth development, the proximity of the dental structures to the irradiated area, and the degree to which these structures are shielded. Contingent on the foregoing, there may be no interference with tooth development, or there may be failure of root formation, dwarfing of the crown or root, or complete absence of development. Fully developed teeth may undergo circumferential cervical destruction as an indirect result of extensive irradiation of the head-and-neck region.

(Top) This 12-year-old patient received x-ray radiation for treatment of a hemangioma of the cheek at the time of development of the teeth. The skin of the face shows a characteristic "orange-peel" appearance over the field of direct irradiation. There is a failure of development of the left side of the face and jaws which is more apparent when the mouth is closed.

(Center) Radiograph of the left side of the maxilla in the same patient. The roots of the premolars and 1st molar have failed to form. The crown of the 2nd premolar is abnormally small.

(Bottom) Heavy therapeutic doses of radiant energy directed in the region of the salivary glands may lead to their atrophy if they are not adequately shielded. The resultant xerostomia and qualitative changes in the saliva probably are the cause of rampant cervical destruction of the teeth in such patients. These rampant lesions of dental caries may lead to "amputation" of the crown. Extraction of teeth from jaws that have been heavily irradiated is contraindicated, so that extraction of teeth before irradiation may be necessary. Daily applications of topical flourides and a strict oral hygiene regimen can aid in preventing the development of radiation caries.

RADIATION EFFECT, SOFT TISSUE AND BONE

Ionizing radiation is of value in treating neoplasms because it injures cells. In the killing of malignant cells, unless the tumor is exceptionally radiosensitive, some degree of injury to normal tissue occurs. The undesirable effects accompanying radiation therapy are related to the type of radiation, the dosage, the division of the dosage, the amount of shielding, and the susceptibility of the individual. Cells may be killed or their functions may be impaired, intercellular substance may degenerate, blood vessels may sclerose or become telangiectatic. There is no immediate indication of damage to skin or mucous membranes. It is only after a period of approximately 2 wk that evidence of injury is apparent. The acute reaction following this latent period consists of redness and edema of the area involved. If the dosage is not too great, this reaction will subside, and the tissues eventually become relatively normal. When tissue is exposed to excessive radiation, progressive degenerative changes occur over a period of years, and carcinoma may develop.

(Top) An inflamed pseudomembranous area is apparent in the vestibular mucosa. This acute radiation reaction occurred 21 days after the institution of x-ray radiation for treatment of carcinoma on the tonsillar pillar.

(Center) This is a section of mucous membrane that had been injured by ionizing radiation. The covering epithelium on the upper border of the photomicrograph is necrotic. There is homogenization of the collagen in the upper lamina propria, and mucoid degeneration is apparent near the lower border of the picture.

(Bottom) Six years before this picture was taken the patient was treated through the right cheek for intraoral carcinoma by x-ray radiation. The residual effects of the radiation are demonstrated by the zone of depigmentation in the lateral aspect of the face and upper neck. In the depigmented area there is also atrophy of the skin with a loss of secondary skin structures. Typical spiderlike, telangiectatic vessels are apparent just anterior to the ear.

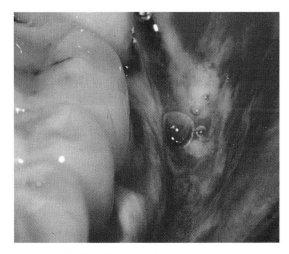

Acute Radiation Reaction, Mucous Membrane

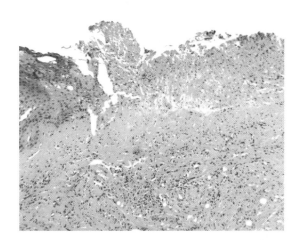

Radiation Effect, Mucous Membrane   ×90

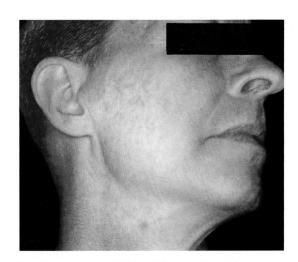

Depigmentation of Skin Following Radiation

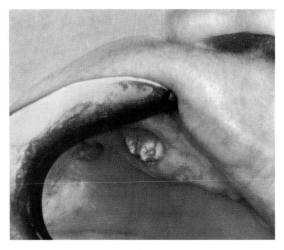

Osteoradionecrosis, Maxilla

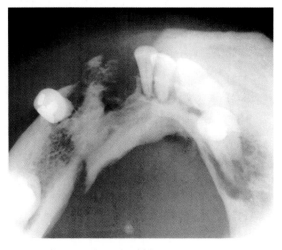

Osteoradionecrosis, Mandible

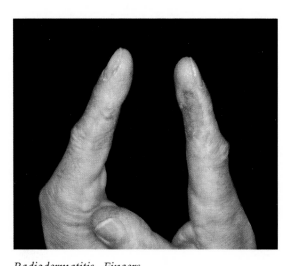

Radiodermatitis, Fingers

RADIATION EFFECT, SOFT TISSUE AND BONE *(continued)*

(Top) When bone is heavily irradiated, its blood vessels may become sclerosed with a resultant impairment of the blood supply and reduced vitality. Such bone may be asymptomatic for years if the overlying mucosa is intact or if it is not injured. The partially devitalized bone has markedly reduced resistance to infection and poor healing power. Thus, trauma or surgical procedures followed by infection may result in extensive, progressive osteomyelitis that will not respond to the usual therapeutic procedures. This particular form of postirradiation osteomyelitis often is called *osteoradionecrosis.* Some authorities prefer to reserve that term for aseptic necrosis of bone following irradiation, using the designation *radiation osteitis* when infection intervenes. The patient has had heavy irradiation of the maxilla followed by osteoradionecrosis. (See p. 104 for the effect of radiation on teeth.)

(Center) This patient had received intensive x-ray radiation for an intraoral carcinoma and remained asymptomatic for years until after extraction of an anterior mandibular tooth. Healing did not occur, and progressive, painful necrosis of the mandible developed. Because periodontal and periapical infections produce bone changes and initiate osteoradionecrosis, the teeth are critical when radiation therapy is to be used in the head and neck region (see p. 104). When intensive radiation is contemplated and the jawbones and salivary glands cannot be shielded adequately, carious and periodontally involved teeth should be extracted prior to irradiation. Extraction of teeth from heavily irradiated bone should be avoided, but if extraction is essential, pre- and postoperative antibiotic therapy, hyperbaric oxygen, and preventive dental therapy may reduce the hazard of osteoradionecrosis.

(Bottom) Fingers of a 50-year-old dentist who, early in practice, had exposed them to an excessive amount of radiation by holding periapical films in patients' mouths. Several years after discontinuing this habit the skin of the fingers gradually became tense, dry, and atrophic. Hyperkeratotic and ulcerative lesions appeared. Skin from the right index finger was removed, and the area was grafted. The lesion was a squamous cell carcinoma.

SOLAR CHEILOSIS

(Top) The degenerative changes in the vermilion portion of the lips of this patient are associated with exposure to the elements, mainly the ultraviolet rays of the sun. The lips, which are covered by a thin, white, keratotic film, have an atrophic appearance. Numerous red, pinpoint erosive areas are present in the exposed portion of the lower lip. Solar cheilosis occurs most frequently in fair-skinned individuals, especially redheads. In advanced cases vermilionectomy is advisable, for this condition predisposes to carcinoma. Treatment in cases of mild involvement consists of applying sunblocking agents to prevent further degenerative changes.

DRUG IDIOSYNCRASY

Certain individuals react to drugs and metals differently than do the majority of persons. Such reactions in the oral cavity are termed *contact stomatitis* if due to direct contact with a drug, or *stomatitis medicamentosa* if the offending agent has been used systemically.

(Center) Marked redness of the oral mucosa is sharply limited to the area in contact with an acrylic partial denture. The denture was strapped to the patient's arm below the axilla, and erythema was present in the contact area within 24 hr. Such contact sensitivity is rare, and the diagnosis should not be made unless a patch test on the skin or mucosa is positive. Scrapings from the suspected denture are adequate for the test. Some patients may react to metals in alloys used for restorations. Inflammation beneath dentures usually results from poor oral hygiene or mechanical irritation (see p. 94) rather than from such sensitivity.

(Bottom) A common oral change related to antibiotic therapy is an extensive black or yellow coating of the tongue. This coating usually does not develop unless the drug has been used for at least a week. It generally persists for several days and then frequently desquamates, leaving the tongue red and sore. The excessive tongue coating is not caused by hypersensitivity but is related to the predominance of fungi in the oral flora. When the flora again becomes balanced, the tongue returns to normal. The patient shown received chloromycetin for 3 wk, at the end of which time the coat was uniform over the entire dorsal surface. The picture was taken a week later, after some desquamation had occurred.

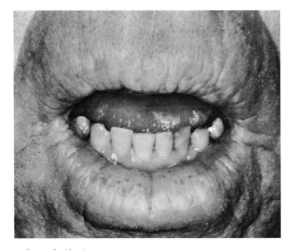

Solar Cheilosis

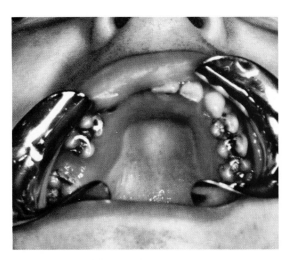

Contact Stomatitis, Acrylic Material

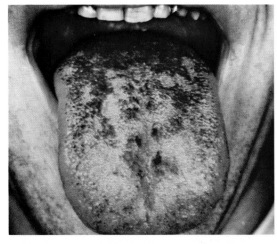

Hairy Tongue Associated with Antibiotic Therapy

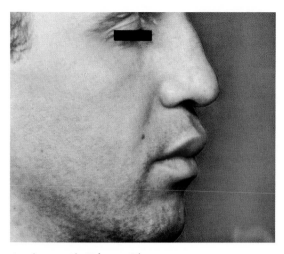

Angioneurotic Edema, Lip

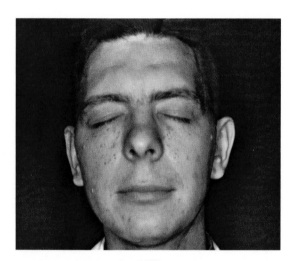

Contact Dermatitis, Penicillin

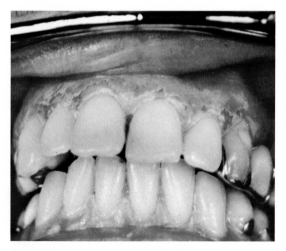

Stomatitis Medicamentosa, Pyridium

DRUG IDIOSYNCRASY *(continued)*

(Top) Marked enlargement of the upper lip is caused by a localized vascular change which allowed the escape of an excessive amount of fluid into the tissue. The patient experienced this reaction each time a local anesthetic was administered. Angioneurotic edema may also occur in individuals who are sensitive to other drugs or to various cosmetics or foods. This type of reaction is most common in the cheeks, lips, and eyelids. The swelling usually does not last longer than 1 or 2 days. It may be reduced by the administration of adrenalin or antihistamines, but ordinarily this is not necessary. With severe laryngeal edema, tracheotomy may be necessary.

(Center) A few drops of penicillin solution accidentally splashed on this dentist's face while giving an injection to a patient. This individual normally has a slender face, but here the cheeks are swollen, the nose and upper lip are enlarged, and the upper eyelids are puffy and red. The presence of papular lesions is also apparent on the cheeks. The picture was taken 36 hr after contact with the drug. This dentist also experiences a severe reaction to the parenteral administration of penicillin.

(Bottom) Stomatitis medicamentosa that followed by 48 hr the administration of Pyridium (phenazopyridine HCL) for an infection of the urinary tract. Swelling, superficial necrosis, and ulceration of the gingiva are seen. The buccal mucosa and pharynx were similarly affected, and the patient complained of intense pain. The stomatitis subsided spontaneously within a few days after discontinuing the use of the drug.

Any drug may cause abnormal reactions in susceptible individuals. Certain groups of drugs, however, such as the antibiotics, sulfonamides, barbiturates, halogens, and salicylates, are responsible for the majority of unusual reactions. Drug idiosyncrasy should always be considered in the differential diagnosis of oral lesions. In some instances the substances responsible for the undesirable effects are ascertained readily, but usually considerable questioning, testing, and elimination of suspicious substances are necessary to determine the offending agent.

MUCOSAL WHITE PATCHES

(LEUKOPLAKIA)

There is much confusion concerning the use of the term *leukoplakia*. Some use it as a clinical term to designate a white plaque in accordance with the primary meaning of the word; others use it to mean a lesion with certain histologic features such as hyperorthokeratosis or dysplasia (dyskeratosis). While these differences in viewpoint cannot be settled arbitrarily, it is highly important that the therapist and the diagnostician thoroughly understand each other's use of the term in any specific case. Since *hyperorthokeratosis, hyperparakeratosis, dyskeratosis,* and *acanthosis* are identified histologically rather than clinically, these terms will be reserved in this Atlas for histologically recognized entities, and the term leukoplakia, or white patch, will be applied arbitrarily to a white, opaque, leathery-appearing plaque not identifiable clinically as some other white lesion (such as lichen planus, drug burn, solar cheilosis, white spongy nevus, carcinoma, etc.). If the lesion shows hyperorthokeratosis, dyskeratosis, or other changes histologically, they will be so designated in the laboratory diagnosis. The irritations that produce white patches may also be contributing factors to carcinoma, and in this sense all white patches should be viewed with some concern by the clinician. The degree of actual cellular change toward malignancy will be indicated by the microscopic appearance of the tissue and will serve as a more definitive guide to the therapist.

(Top) White lesion on the ventral tongue that on biopsy proved to be hyperorthokeratosis.

(Center) A diffuse area of leukoplakia in the buccal mucosa of a tobacco chewer. The pouch created by the wad of tobacco is apparent opposite the maxillary molar region. The involved area is soft and pliable, and a biopsy revealed only increased surface keratinization.

(Bottom) A very thick, extensive area of leukoplakia in the mandibular alveolar mucosa. The clinical appearance may suggest carcinoma, but histologic examination showed it to be benign hyperorthokeratosis.

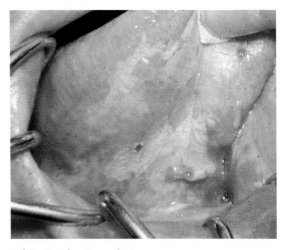

White Patch, Ventral Tongue

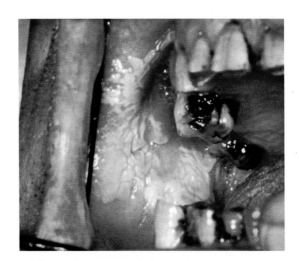

White Patch, Hyperorthokeratosis

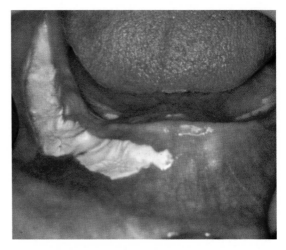

White Patch, Hyperorthokeratosis

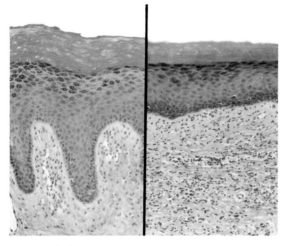

Hyperorthokeratosis   × 90

MUCOSAL WHITE PATCHES *(continued)*

(Top)   In the photomicrograph at the left, which is a section of a white patch, it is apparent that the epithelium, except for a heavy layer of orthokeratin, varies little from normal (see p. 2.) The epithelial cells stain uniformly and do not vary in size and shape. There is little, if any, interference with their orderly maturation. Because of the degree of surface keratinization it is evident that this lesion would have appeared clinically as a very thick white patch. The photomicrograph on the right, a portion of another white patch, reveals a heavy layer of orthokeratin. The flattening of the rete pegs suggest epithelial atrophy.

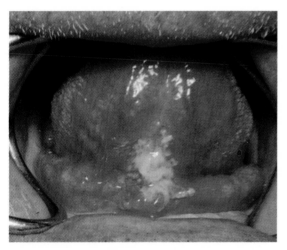

White Patch, Mild Dysplasia

(Center)   The white lesion in this case is thick, extensive, leathery, and fissured. Histologic examination revealed epithelial alterations which suggested future carcinomatous change (mild dysplasia). The question of which white patches should be biopsied is often asked. Histologic examination should be made of all such lesions that persist after removal of local irritants unless there is absolutely no doubt of the diagnosis. Occasionally the most innocent-looking white area is found to have malignant potentialities when examined microscopically. Even individuals with extensive clinical experience frequently do not rely on clinical evaluation alone.

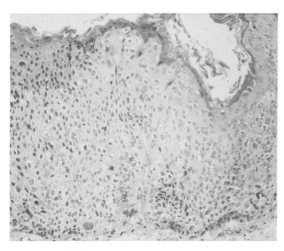

Severe Dysplasia   × 180

(Bottom)   Epithelial changes suggestive of premalignancy are hyperchromatism, loss of polarity, increase in number of mitotic figures, and irregularity of size and shape of nuclei. These changes are implied in the term *malignant dyskeratosis,* although literally dyskeratosis signifies only disordered keratin formation. Probably *dysplasia* is the better term. In the specimen illustrated there are many hyperchromatic cells in the basal layer and a loss of cellular polarity. Cells with abnormal shapes (pleomorphism) and several mitotic figures are evident in the middle layers. These changes are sufficient to warn of possible progression to malignancy.

(Top) Histologic examination shows an extreme degree of keratinization, a prominent granular layer, a disorderly arrangement of cells in the malpighian layer (cellular atypia), and an irregular downward proliferation of the rete pegs. The basal layer is somewhat difficult to identify because of its invasion by inflammatory cells. Irregularly shaped cells with hyperchromatic nuclei (better seen at higher magnification) are present in the lower layers of the epithelium. Cellular atypias may remain static for long periods or progress to severe dysplasia or carcinoma in situ. Lesions with this diagnosis should be followed carefully. A change in the clinical appearance should alert the clinician to the need for rebiopsy.

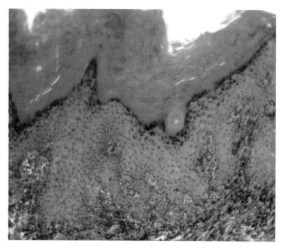

Marked Hyperorthokeratosis With Some Cellular Atypia × 80

NICOTINIC STOMATITIS

(Center) In this moderately advanced case of nicotinic stomatitis, numerous red dots—the inflamed and dilated orifices of salivary gland ducts—are apparent throughout the whitened palatal mucosa. Earlier the mucosa is intensely red; later it becomes pale, due to a slight increase in keratinization. In advanced cases the palatal tissue is more heavily keratinized, and nodules appear. A few of these nodules (which are related to hyperplasia of the underlying glands, to retention of saliva, and to fibrosis) are seen in this case in the middle palatal region. Nicotinic stomatitis is observed most frequently in pipe smokers but does occur in individuals who use cigars or cigarettes. The mucosal changes are caused by heat and the irritating effect of the combustion products of tobacco. The intensity of these changes is dependent on the manner of smoking, the quantity of tobacco used, and the sensitivity of the individual.

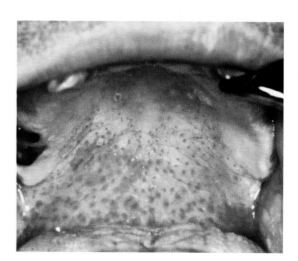

Nicotinic Stomatitis

(Bottom) Numerous umbilicated nodules, typical of an advanced case, are evident in the posterior gland-bearing areas. The entire palatal mucosa, except under the partial denture, has a white, cooked appearance. Irritating effects of smoking may be reduced under dental appliances covering the palate. Nicotinic stomatitis is a definite clinical entity. The histologic findings, though not pathognomonic, include hyperplasia of surface epithelium with deep, broad, fused rete pegs; hyperorthokeratosis; dilatation of gland ducts; squamous metaplasia of the ductal epithelium; and sialadentis of minor glands.

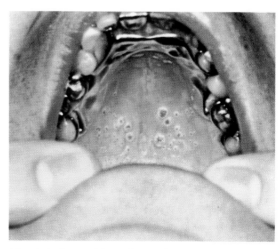

Nicotinic Stomatitis, Advanced Stage

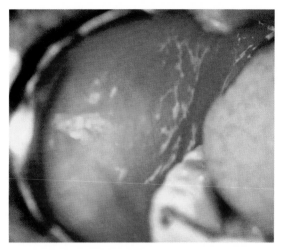

Lichen Planus, Buccal Mucosa, Lacelike Pattern

papule

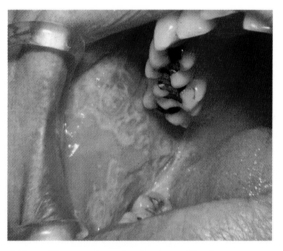

Lichen Planus, Annular Lesions, Cheek

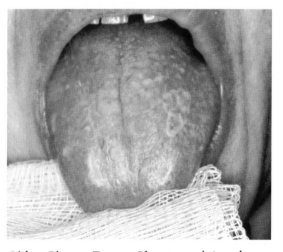

Lichen Planus, Tongue, Plaques, and Annular Lesions

LICHEN PLANUS

Lichen planus is an inflammatory dermatosis, which also involves mucous membranes, characterized by keratotic lesions of various patterns. The etiology is not known, but the disease is often associated with some degree of emotional tension. Lichen planus is an annoying but not a serious affliction, and the lesions frequently regress when the emotional state of the patient improves. Oral manifestations may occur alone, or they may precede, accompany, or follow cutaneous lesions.

(Top) In the buccal mucosa are several interlacing fine white lines. Small raised dots mark the intersections of the lines. When lesions present a clinical appearance such as this, the diagnosis need not be presumptive, and a biopsy is unnecessary. Not all lesions of lichen planus are as typical as the ones shown here. There may be extensive white plaques, nodules, and erosions. However, careful examination of the lesions may reveal Wickham's striae, which should suggest the diagnosis of lichen planus. The appearance of lesions is sometimes altered by cheek chewing, a habit not uncommon in individuals with this disease.

(Center) The oral eruption, which occurs most frequently in the buccal mucosa, tongue, and lower lip, usually is characterized by slightly raised, white, fine dots and thin lines (Wickham's Striae). In this illustration keratotic lines form the typical lacy pattern of lichen planus opposite the maxillary molars while a white plaque, which also may be a manifestation of lichen planus, is seen opposite the mandibular molars. One must evaluate the total appearance of lesions in suspected lichen planus.

(Bottom) Extensive keratinization on the dorsal surface of the tongue, producing a white plaque. On the left side of the tongue, however, there are annular lesions, posterior to which are discrete white dots, and in other areas a few thin, white lines may be seen. The presence of more characteristic lesions elsewhere in the oral cavity may help the differential diagnosis. In case of doubt, a biopsy is indicated.

(Top)   Lichen planus of the gingiva is not common. The erosive type, as shown here, must be distinguished from desquamative gingivitis. The presence or absence of Wickham's striae may help differentiate the two diseases. Erosive lesions occurring elsewhere in the oral cavity may at times closely resemble ulcerated lesions of lupus erythematosus, as fine white lines may also be associated with the latter. Erosive lesions of lichen planus are sometimes painful, but the nonerosive manifestations are symptomless. Lesions of this disease occurring in other mucous membranes are similar to those found in the oral cavity.

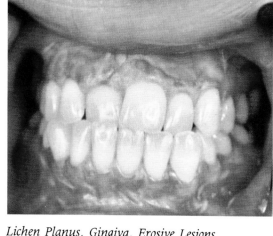

Lichen Planus, Gingiva, Erosive Lesions

(Center)   Cutaneous lesions of lichen planus may be generalized but are usually confined to a few areas, often symmetrically distributed. The flexor surfaces of the wrist, forearm, and lower leg are the sites most frequently involved. The eruption, often pruritic, begins as very small, flat-topped, round, or angulated papules covered by a thin, horny film. These enlarge and may coalesce. They have a glistening surface, and close inspection will reveal small white raised dots and linear streaks. The early lesions may be purplish red, while the older ones exhibit a light-violet hue. Brown macules, which are due to the presence of numerous melanophages in the upper dermis, often mark the site of healed lesions.

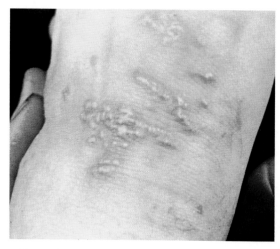

Lichen Planus, Cutaneous Lesions

(Bottom)   The histologic features of lichen planus, as shown in the accompanying biopsy specimen from the buccal mucosa, include: (1) an infiltration of lymphocytes in intimate relation to the epithelium and sharply limited to the upper lamina propria; (2) liquefaction degeneration of the basal layer; (3) saw-toothed rete pegs; (4) prominent granular layer; and (5) a moderate degree of hyperorthokeratosis. Lesions in the oral mucosa often show no granular layer, and parakeratin may be formed rather than orthokeratin. In the hypertrophic form of the disease there is considerable hyperplasia of the epithelium and an excessive amount of keratin. In the atrophic type the covering epithelium is thin, and the rete pegs are flattened.

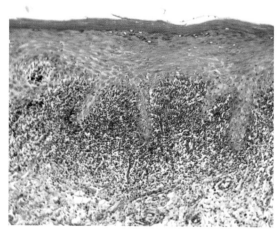

Lichen Planus, Oral Biopsy Specimen   × 80

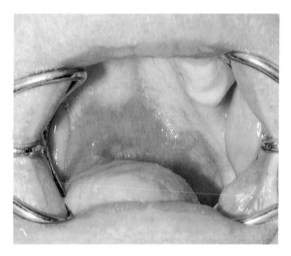

Erythroplakia, Soft Palate

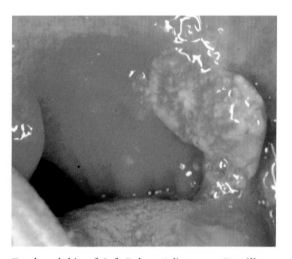

Erythroplakia of Soft Palate Adjacent to Tonsillar Carcinoma

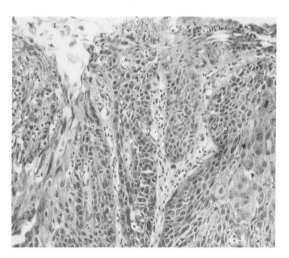

Carcinoma in situ ×950

MUCOSAL RED PATCHES

(ERYTHROPLAKIA)

The term *erythroplakia (erythroplasia)* is applied to noninflammatory red velvety areas of the oral mucosa that are frequently asymptomatic. Studies have shown that only about 4% of leukoplakic lesions develop into cancer in 20 years. In contrast over 60% of erythroplakic lesions show invasive carcinoma or *in situ* changes at the time they are seen clinically and biopsied. Some lesions of erythroplakia may be granular or speckled with white dots. A high level of suspicion for red lesions of the oral mucosa, early establishment of diagnosis, and proper treatment are important to increase survival rates and quality of life for those with these potentially life-threatening lesions.

(Top) The majority of erythroplakic lesions occur in the floor of the mouth or on the soft palate complex. Any persistent (14 days or more) asymptomatic erythroplakic lesion in high-risk patients (smokers and drinkers) should be viewed with great suspicion and biopsied. This velvety red area on the palate proved to be carcinoma *in situ*.

(Center) Erythroplakia is now considered to be the earliest and most predominant sign of oral cancer. It is frequently asymptomatic. If treatment, either by surgery or radiation, as was done in this case on the soft palate and tonsil, is accomplished prior to metastases developing, an excellent survival rate may be achieved.

(Bottom) Photomicrograph of erythroplakic lesion. The histology is carcinoma *in situ*. These lesions present a red appearance clinically because they are devoid of surface keratin and have dilated capillaries in the subjacent connective tissue. If not removed this lesion can be expected to progress to full-blown carcinoma.

GEOGRAPHIC TONGUE

(BENIGN MIGRATORY GLOSSITIS)

(Top) This disease is characterized by migrating circinate or ovoid inflammatory lesions on the dorsum of the tongue. These lesions, which arise without apparent cause, are red and slightly depressed and have a grayish-yellow border. The redness is related to loss of filiform papillae, desquamation of the superficial prickle cells, and hyperemia. Careful examination of a lesion usually will reveal that there is some regeneration of filiform papillae centrally, and that the redness is more intense near the periphery. Patients may complain of a slight burning sensation, but usually the lesions are painless. Similar lesions occurring on the lips and buccal mucosa have been reported as *migratory stomatitis*. The degree of migration varies with the case; in some instances the lesions remain relatively static for weeks, while in others evidence of wandering is apparent every few days. There may be periods when the tongue is completely healed. This disease may persist for years, and satisfactory treatment is unknown. It is of no significance, but patients may need to be continually reassured of its innocuousness.

(Center) Near the center of the upper border is the raised periphery of a lesion. This area is characterized by parakeratosis; epithelial hyperplasia; long, broad, fused rete pegs; edema of the upper malpighian layer; and a heavy infiltration of neutrophils. To the left of this raised area is normal tongue mucosa, and to the right (red area clinically) there is desquamation of the epithelial cells. Further to the right, beyond the scope of this photomicrograph, was severe desquamation, with only thin epithelial plates remaining over the extremely vascular connective tissue papillae.

BLACK HAIRY TONGUE

(Bottom) Black hairy tongue (lingua nigra) is the name applied to a condition in which the filiform papillae are so greatly elongated that they somewhat resemble hairs. The "hairs" may become stained by food, tobacco, or chromogenic microorganisms. Hairy tongue may develop following the use of various chemotherapeutic agents. (see p. 107.) It also may occur without apparent cause, and in these cases tends to be persistent.

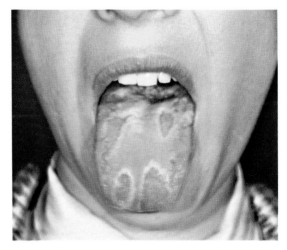

Geographic Tongue

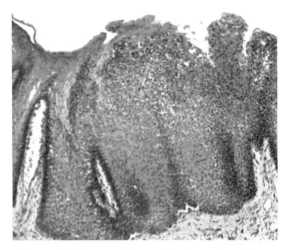

Geographic Tongue, Biopsy Specimen from Edge of Lesion ×75

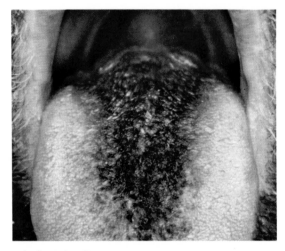

Black Hairy Tongue

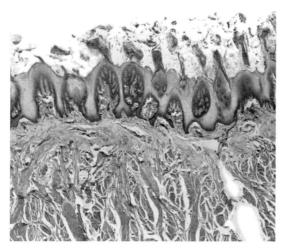

Black Hairy Tongue   × 15

BLACK HAIRY TONGUE *(continued)*

(Top)   Biopsy specimen from an individual with a persistent hairy tongue. At intervals along the upper surface are long projections of keratin that are hyperplastic filiform papillae. Desquamated keratin and other debris may be seen between the papillae. Compare with normal filiform papillae, page 5. Gently stroking from posterior to anterior with a tongue blade two or three times daily will help to reduce black hairy tongue.

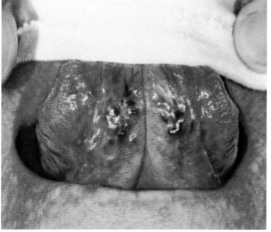

Lingual Varicosities

VARICOSE VEINS, TONGUE

(Center)   Purplish-blue nodular areas on the ventral surface of the tongue. These varicosities (oral phlebectasia) are due to dilatation and increased tortuosity of the lingual veins. Dilated veins in this location are not uncommon in older individuals. They are probably of no clinical significance. In general, varicosities are related to increased venous pressure, weakness of the vein wall, and lack of support by surrounding tissue. Complications such as ulceration, thrombosis, and hemorrhage arising as a result of lingual varicosities are very rare. The patient should be advised of their innocuous nature.

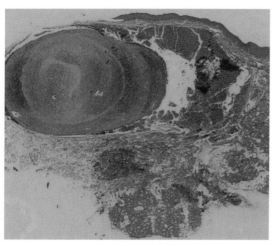

Lingual Varicosity   × 4

(Bottom)   Photomicrograph of lingual varicosity. A large dilated thin-walled vein is present in the center of the specimen just below the surface epithelium. A thrombus occupies the right portion of the varicosity. Thrombi are rare in lingual varicosities. Below and to the left is normal accessory salivary gland tissue.

2. CONDITIONS RESULTING FROM ALTERED IMMUNE STATES

RECURRENT APHTHOUS ULCERS

(CANKER SORES)

Recurrent aphthous ulcers (RAU) are common oral lesions that sometimes present problems in differential diagnosis and are frustrating to treat and manage.

(Top) This gingival ulcer is characteristic of RAU. It is superficial and has a yellowish, fibrinous base. The red, inflamed border is irregular. RAU are characterized by intense pain. They persist for up to 14 days and may be multiple.

The etiology is multifactorial. The immune system seems actively involve in reaction to bacterial and autoimmune antigens, resulting in focal tissue necrosis and ulcer formation. A number of precipitating factors have been identified, including minor trauma, stress, subclinical systemic disease, and nutritional deficiencies. Systemic and topical steroid applications tend to decrease the duration and severity of RAU but have no effect on the recurrence rate.

MAJOR APHTHAE

Periadenitis Mucosa Necrotica Recurrens

(SCARRING APHTHAE)

Major aphthous ulcers occur as large painful ulcers, which may persist for as long as 6 weeks and leave a scar upon healing. Scarring usually is evident in areas where there have been repeated lesions. Patients with PMNR may be poorly nourished because the pain associated with the ulcers makes it difficult to eat. The disorder occurs in gland-bearing areas of the mucosa. Histologically, it is characterized by necrosis and inflammation in the region of the ducts of the minor salivary glands. The cause is probably an altered immune response. Treatment with steroids may offer relief.

(Center) On the lower lip near the corner of the mouth is a large, well-developed, depressed ulcer that is characteristic of this disease. It has begun to heal, and some fibrosis has occurred, as evidenced by the elevated tissue at the periphery of the lesion.

(Bottom) This patient was afflicted with scarring aphthae for 20 years. In the vestibular mucosa near the commissure are numerous firm, irregular elevations. These are fibrotic areas associated with the healing of ulcers that have formed repeatedly in this location.

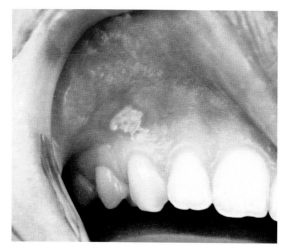

Recurrent Aphthous Ulcer, Gingiva

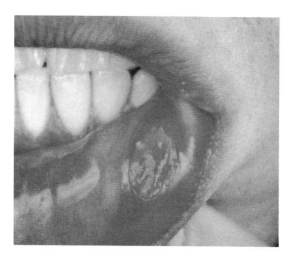

Periadenitis Mucosa Necrotica Recurrens

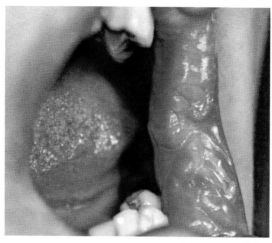

Periadenitis Mucosa Necrotica Recurrens, Scarring

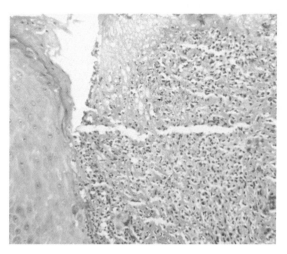

Aphthous Ulcer × 40

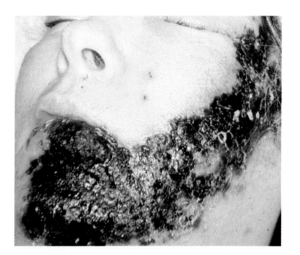

Herpes Zoster

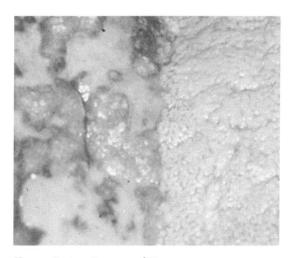

Herpes Zoster, Dorsum of Tongue

MAJOR APHTHAE *(continued)*

(Top) Biopsy specimen from an aphthous ulcer. The intact surface oral epithelium is seen at the right. The ulcerated surface, at the left, is covered with precipitated fibrin in which are entrapped numerous inflammatory cells. This covering of precipitated fibrin appears clinically as a greyish pseudomembrane over the surface of an aphthous ulcer.

HERPES ZOSTER

Herpes zoster is most likely to occur in older individuals or in those who are immunosuppressed either by cancer therapy or who have Hodgkin's disease. It is also a complication in patients who are immunosuppressed because of AIDS (p. 121).

(Center) The varicella-zoster (VZ) virus causes an acute primary infection (chickenpox). Following recovery from the primary episode, the virus becomes latent in sensory ganglia. Reactivation results in zoster or shingles along the sensory distribution of the affected nerve, in this case the maxillary and mandibular divisions of the trigeminal ganglion in this patient with lymphocytic leukemia.

(Bottom) Like the skin lesions, the intraoral lesions of zoster are unilateral and may sharply demarcate the sensory distribution of the affected nerve. Because of the seriousness of the infection in immunocompromised hosts, vigorous treatment may be necessary. Acyclovir and adenine arabinoside have shown some promise in controlling these lesions.

SJÖGREN'S SYNDROME

This syndrome is characterized by salivary gland swelling, involvement of the lacrimal glands, keratoconjunctivitis, and rheumatoid arthritis. Patients complain of dry mouth and eyes. It is more frequent in females than in males.

(Top) This patient exhibited the typical symptoms of the syndrome: involvement of the salivary glands, dryness of the eyes and mouth extending to the nares and pharynx, and rheumatoid arthritis. Her serum immunoglobulin levels were elevated.

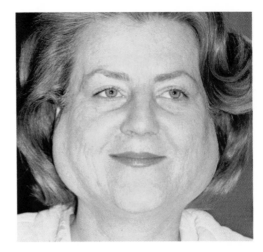

Sjögren's Syndrome

(Center) Severe dryness of the ocular mucosa due to lacrimal gland involvement results in dryness of the conjunctiva and some keratinization of the conjunctival mucosa (keratoconjunctivitis sicca). Soreness and inflammation occur (xerophthalmia) because the natural lubricating effect of tears is absent. Treatment of the oral and ocular dryness is symptomatic. Artificial saliva and artificial tears are recommended.

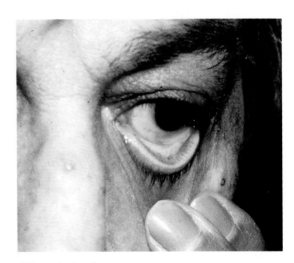

Sjögren's Syndrome

(Bottom) Biopsy of the greatly enlarged parotid gland from the patient shown at top of page revealed heavy infiltration with lymphocytes, obliterating all the functional salivary gland tissue. A few scattered islands of squamous and ductal epithelium were observed among the numerous lymphocytes. This feature gives rise to the term *benign lymphoepithelial lesion,* which is sometimes applied to the microscopic appearance in cases of Sjögren's syndrome and Mikulicz's disease.

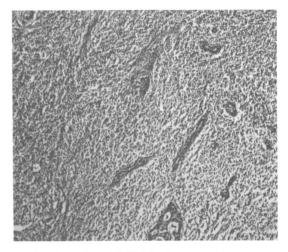

Benign Lymphoepithelial Lesion ×40

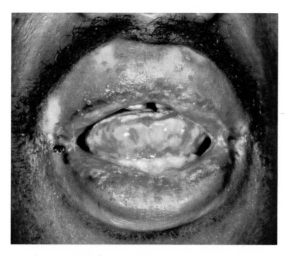

Erythema Multiforme, Tongue and Lip Lesions

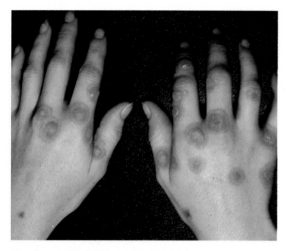

Erythema Multiforme, Target Lesions

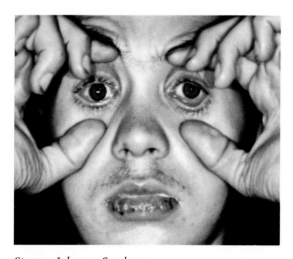

Stevens-Johnson Syndrome

ERYTHEMA MULTIFORME

Erythema multiforme is an acute inflammatory disease of unknown cause that is characterized by a variety of cutaneous and mucosal lesions. These lesions may be macular, papular, vesicular, or bullous. The disease usually runs a course of from 10 to 20 days and tends to recur. The features of the disorder suggest a transient autoimmune defect which may be triggered by antigens and other factors. In the oral cavity there often are extensive, superficially ulcerated, irregular red lesions that are sometimes covered by a grayish-yellow exudate. The whole oral and pharyngeal mucosa may be involved, making eating and swallowing most difficult. In severe cases there is often a sharp rise in temperature, headache, and malaise, and the patient may be acutely ill for 3 or 4 days. Stevens-Johnson syndrome is a variety of erythema multiforme in which there are oral and ocular lesions, fever, and severe constitutional symptoms. In some instances of erythema multiforme there may be a concomitant gynecomastia. Administration of steroids appears to shorten the course of the disease and reduce the symptoms.

(Top) The entire tongue is raw and red, and a grayish pseudomembrane is apparent in several areas. The lip lesions, which are nearly healed here, tend to be covered with a hemorrhagic crust. The chief complaint, even in cases with extensive cutaneous manifestations, usually is related to the painful oral lesions. The treatment consists of administering steroids and relieving symptoms. A bland mouthwash is indicated, and systemic use of broad-spectrum antibiotics is useful in combating secondary infection. In some instances intravenous feeding is necessary.

(Center) "Target" lesions on the skin are characteristic of erythema multiforme.

(Bottom) Stevens-Johnson syndrome in a young adult. Conjunctivitis, sialorrhea, and crusted lip lesions are apparent. The patient also had extensive intraoral lesions, fever, and leukopenia.

ACQUIRED IMMUNODEFICIENCY SYNDROME (AIDS)

Acquired immunodeficiency syndrome (AIDS) is a disease caused by the human immunodeficiency virus (HIV). HIV may live in the human body for years before actual signs or symptoms appear. Because of depressed immunity, individuals become susceptible to a variety of other diseases. Patients with AIDS and AIDS-related complex (ARC) require dental care, and it is the responsibility of the dental profession to provide this care. The use of appropriate barrier technics when examining or treating dental patients is strongly recommended by the Centers for Disease Control and the ADA. Patients with AIDS or ARC may exhibit Kaposi's sarcoma, hairy leukoplakia, HIV-gingivitis and candidiasis, These patients are at high risk for a variety of other conditions including non-Hodgkin's lymphoma (see p. 175), recurrent herpes, aphthous ulcers (see p. 117), squamous cell carcinoma (see p. 168), herpes zoster (see p. 118), papillary lesions including veruccae and condylomata (see p. 88), and a variety of bacterial, viral, and fungal infections.

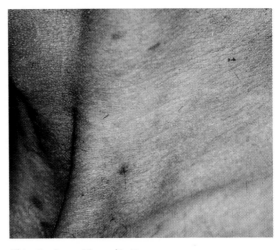

Skin Lesions, Kaposi's Sarcoma

(Top)   Kaposi's sarcoma (KS) occurring on the skin of the neck in an AIDS patient. They also occur frequently on the trunk and arms as well as the head and neck area.

(Center)   Kaposi's sarcoma of the palate. Early lesions are flat, later stages are lobulated. Greenspan and Greenspan report that among homosexual men with KS, 51% had oral lesions.

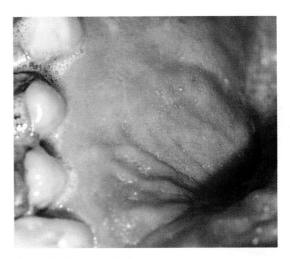

Kaposi's Sarcoma, Palate

(Bottom)   Photomicrograph of biopsy of KS. There is a spindle cell pattern with associated red blood cell extravasation. Two cells in the early stage of mitosis can be identified.

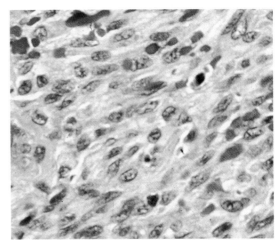

Kaposi's Sarcoma   ×40

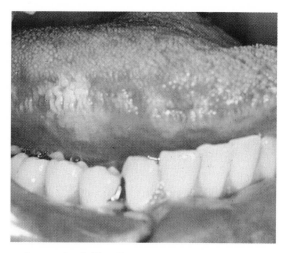

Hairy Leukoplakia, Tongue

ACQUIRED IMMUNODEFICIENCY SYNDROME (AIDS) *(continued)*

(Top)   Hairy leukoplakia (HL) is a frequent and early clinical sign of exposure to HIV. The majority of patients do not have AIDS at the time of diagnosis of HL, but AIDS later develops in a high proportion of patients. Clinically the lesions of HL develop on the lateral/ventral aspects of the tongue in homosexual males. The patients report no symptoms.

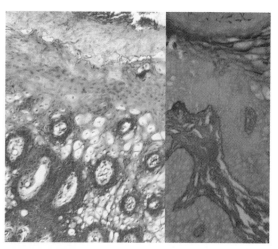

*Hairy Leukoplakia, H & E (left)
and PAS (right)   × 40*

(Center)   Microscopically, HL consists of hyperplastic and hyperparakeratotic epithelium that shows multiple projections. Vacuolated cells with clear cytoplasm and small nuclei surrounded by a halo, resembling *koilocytes* are present in the middle layers of epithelium *(left)*. Special stains reveal the presence of candidal hyphae in the superficial layers *(right)*. Epstein-Barr virus and human papilloma virus have been identified in the vacuolated cells.

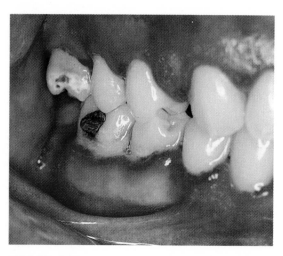

HIV-Gingivitis

(Bottom)   There is an increased frequency and severity of gingival and periodontal disease in HIV-infected homosexual males. Research data suggest that HIV-gingivitis (HIV-G) is frequently seen before a dramatic decrease in T4 lymphocyte numbers occurs. The gingivitis may be followed by a rapidly progressive, painful, and locally destructive disease, HIV-periodontitis (HIV-P). The HIV-gingivitis often exhibits a distinct linear red band, and punctate red lesions of the attached gingiva. Bleeding occurs readily upon probing.

PEMPHIGUS VULGARIS

(Top) Pemphigus vulgaris, an uncommon serious autoimmune disease, is characterized by the formation of intraepithelial bullae in the skin and mucous membrane. Oral lesions may be the first sign of the disease. Intact oral bullae are not commonly seen, for soon after formation they rupture, and much of the collapsed membranous covering is lost, leaving ulcerated areas around which there is little reaction. In this case several collapsed bullae are present on the buccal mucosa. The diagnosis of pemphigus is difficult, and often it must be based at least partially on the clinical course of the disease.

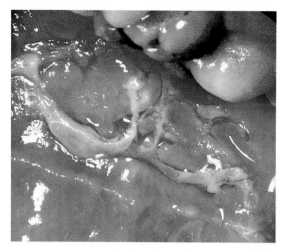

Pemphigus Vulgaris, Oral Lesions

(Center) Photomicrograph of pemphigus lesion. The empty space between the squamous epithelium and the lamina propria is the vesicle and contained fluid. Basal cells remain attached to the connective tissue at the base of the specimen, making this a suprabasilar vesicle. Immunofluorescence reveals intense reactivity at intercellular junctions between epithelial cells.

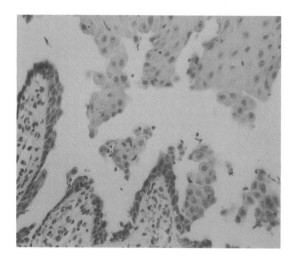

Pemphigus Vulgaris ×40

BENIGN MUCOUS MEMBRANE PEMPHIGOID (BMMP)

(Bottom) Named *pemphigoid* because of its superficial resemblance to pemphigus, BMMP is an autoimmune disease characterized by the formation of vesicles or blisters on cutaneous and mucosal surfaces. Immunofluorescence reveals concentration of immune products associated with the hemidesmosome complex at the epithelial–connective tissue interface. The vesicles are subepithelial. Ruptured vesicles shown here involve the palate and alveolar ridge. Similar involvement of conjunctival mucosa may lead to scarring and blindness. It is more common in older individuals.

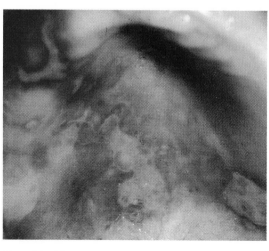

Pemphigoid

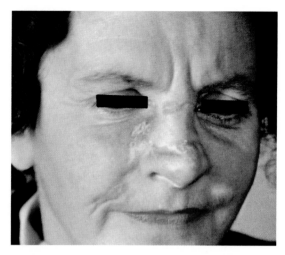

Nonsystemic Lupus Erythematosus, Cutaneous Lesions

LUPUS ERYTHEMATOSUS (LE)

(Top)   Now recognized as an autoimmune disease LE occurs in 2 forms—systemic and chronic discoid (nonsystemic), the latter limited to skin and mucous membranes. The cutaneous eruptions occur due to trauma or solar radiation damage. Antigenic DNA is formed. Immune complexes attract neutrophils, which release lysosomal enzymes, which in turn cause tissue damage. The eruption over the bridge of the nose and zygomatic eminences (butterfly pattern), consists of slightly raised, red patches covered by greasy keratin scales. In the *systemic* form, there are accumulations of immune complexes in numerous organs as well as skin and mucosal lesions. Diagnosis may be established by finding LE cells in peripheral blood or bone marrow.

SCLERODERMA

Diffuse scleroderma is a generalized connective tissue disease that shows some of the immunologic markers of autoimmune diseases. A lymphokine of T-cell origin stimulates fibroblasts to over-produce collagen. The most obvious clinical feature of this disease is stiffening of the skin, although symptoms may be variable and multiple. The scarlike tissue limits motion and may gradually lead to inability to swallow. Skin appendages atrophy; the epidermis becomes thinned and may be hyperpigmented. Vascular lumina may be diminished due to intimal proliferation, and the kidneys, lungs, liver, and muscles may become involved in the fibrosing process. A local form of the disease (circumscribed scleroderma) involves only limited regions of the skin and produces no visceral lesions.

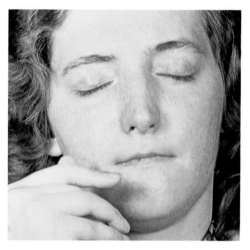

Scleroderma

(Center)   This patient shows the typical picture of moderately advanced scleroderma. The natural lines of the face are nearly obliterated, she has a fixed expression giving her a Mona Lisa-like appearance, and her skin appears somewhat bronzed. The eyelids and fingers, particularly, show the atrophic, shiny appearance that overlies the collagenous changes in the connective tissue. Sclerosed tissue has produced discrete nodules on the eyelids. Because of the rigidity of her sclerosed skin she could not open her mouth wide, and the movement of her fingers was limited.

(Bottom)   In some cases of scleroderma there is a uniform thickening of the periodontal ligament with disorientation of the periodontal fibers about one or more of the teeth—mainly the posteriors. An increase in the width of the lamina dura is often associated with this distinctive change.

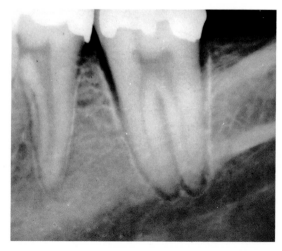

Scleroderma, Wide Periodontal Space About 2nd Molar

V

Non-neoplastic Conditions of the Jaw Bones

INTRODUCTION

The maxilla and mandible are subject to changes as the result of local trauma, radiation, inflammation, and developmental, genetic and systemic influences. Obviously, inflammation of the jaws most frequently is associated with odontogenic infections (see Chapter III).

Bone is the most plastic tissue of the body. During bone growth osteoblastic activity dominates over osteoclastic activity. When bone is being resorbed or undergoing atrophy, osteoclasia becomes more prominent whether the cause is disuse, pressure, inflammation or metabolic or neoplastic activity. During its maintenance period osteoblastic and osteoclastic activities are minimal and equal. These conditions may be illustrated diagramatically as follows:

Osteoblastic activity>osteoclastic activity=growth

i.e., enlargement (p. 127), sclerosis, (p. 140), hyperostosis, (p. 23), acromegaly (p. 137), osteogenic neoplasia (p. 177)

Osteoclastic activity>osteoblastic activity=bone loss

i.e., atrophy (p. 19), giant cell lesion (p. 98), hyperparathryroidism, (p. 136), and osteolytic neoplasia (p. 166).

Osteoblastic activity=osteoclastic activity during maintenance periods.

When osteoblastic and osteoclastic activities are disorganized dysplasia results

i.e., Paget's disease (p. 129)

The jaws are unique in that they contain numerous teeth embedded in bone and extending beyond the body tissues into the oral cavity. This arrangement subjects them to insults from microorganisms, chemical agents, and trauma far beyond that of other bones unless these are subjected to compound fractures or penetration by shrapnel or other objects.

Lesions of the jaws may result in enlargement, sclerosis (with increased radiopacity), or resorption (with increased radiolucency). There may be pain associated with bone lesions, especially those of inflammatory origin.

Radiographic examination is valuable in the diagnosis of osseous conditions but should not be depended upon as the sole method of examination. Clinical examination and history are very important, and in many instances biopsy is essential.

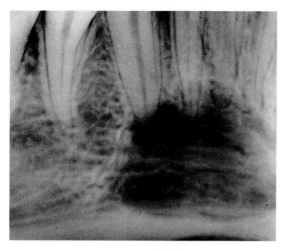

Traumatic Bone Lesion, Mandible

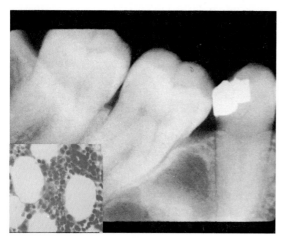

Bone Marrow Defect   Inset × 100

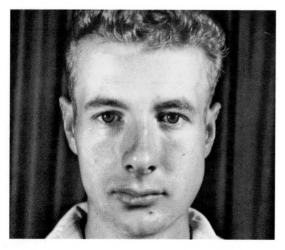

Monostotic Fibrous Dysplasia, Left Mandible

TRAUMATIC BONE LESION

(Top) Traumatic bone lesions (hemorrhagic or extravasation cysts) are localized areas of bone necrosis that are purported to result from intramedullary hematomas that do not become organized. The intraosseous hemorrhage is believed to be related to a traumatic incident in an area of the bone that has hematopoietic marrow. In specific cases, however, a history of trauma may be impossible to obtain. These bone lesions usually are discovered during a routine radiographic examination. They are found most frequently near the apices of teeth but are not related to periapical inflammation. The teeth in the vicinity test vital, and thus these lesions may be differentiated from apical periodontal cysts. Exposure of a traumatic lesion reveals a dry bony cavity containing no cystic lining. The cortical bone over the lesion may be thin but usually is not expanded.

OSTEOPOROTIC BONE MARROW DEFECT

(Center) This condition presents as a focal radiolucency in the jaw, most often in the mandible at the site of a previous extraction. It probably represents normal marrow in an area of bone remodeling or repair. It is usually asymptomatic, discovered on routine radiographic examination. Differential diagnosis includes residual granuloma or cyst, central tumor, and traumatic bone lesion.

FIBROUS DYSPLASIA

Fibrous dysplasia is a skeletal disease characterized by replacement of the bone and bone marrow by a fibrous connective tissue. Numerous irregular and haphazardly arranged osseous spicules develop within the fibrous connective tissue. A polyostotic type of the disease is characterized by fibrous bone lesions that usually are unilateral, brown pigmentation of the skin, precocious puberty (in females), and other endocrine disturbances (Albright's syndrome). The monostotic type shows only the fibrous replacement of bone and bone marrow in a single bone without related endocrine and dermal symptoms. Whether or not the two diseases are related is debatable.

(Bottom) Monostotic fibrous dysplasia in the mandible of a 24-year-old patient. The swelling of the left side of the face, which was asymptomatic, first became noticeable 4 years previously, following the extraction of two lower left molar teeth. Explora-

tion of the lesion revealed that the cortex was very thin but intact, and the interior of the bone was filled with tough, brownish-white, resilient, gritty soft tissue.

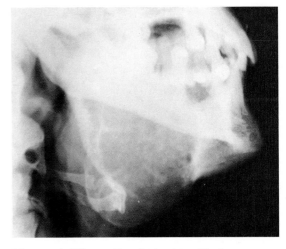

(Top) Radiograph of patient shown on previous page. The mandible shows a diffuse, poorly demarcated, multilocular expansile lesion that involves most of the body of the ramus on one side. The radiographic appearance varies with the stage of the disease, showing more radiolucency early and more radiopacity later. In this case the normal trabecular pattern has been lost, and the cortical layer is poorly defined. There is a ground-glass appearance, suggesting that there has been irregular calcification within the fibrous connective tissue.

Monostotic Fibrous Dysplasia, Mandibular Radiograph

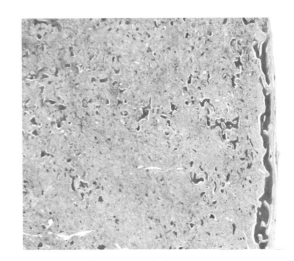

(Center) Low-power view of a section of tissue from the case shown above. The lesion is composed largely of fibrous connective tissue with osteoblastic potential. There are numerous purple-stained spicules of bone scattered through the connective tissue and thin cortical bone at the right margin. The scattered osseous spicules absorb x-rays, causing the ground-glass appearance seen in the radiograph above.

Monostotic Fibrous Dysplasia ×11

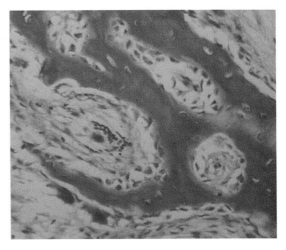

(Bottom) Higher magnification from one area of this case shows irregular C-shaped bone trabeculae and the mesenchymal stroma. As the lesion matures the osteoblastic activity increases, resulting in more bone replacing the matrix and in a greater radiopacity.

Monostotic Fibrous Dysplasia ×100

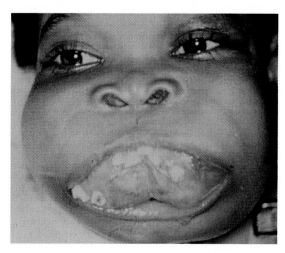

Cherubism

CHERUBISM (FAMILIAL FIBROUS DYSPLASIA)

(Top) Cherubism is characterized by bilateral, painless mandibular (and often corresponding maxillary) swellings that cause a fullness of the cheeks. It has a very early clinical onset, as early as 18 months of age. Maxillary involvement can produce a slight upward turning of the child's eyes, revealing an abnormal amount of sclera. The condition has been termed *familial fibrous dysplasia* because the swelling of the jaws is reminiscent of the swelling that occurs with fibrous dysplasia of bone. The two conditions are not related, however. Studies have shown that cherubism is inherited, most likely as an autosomal dominant condition. There is variable expressivity between generations.

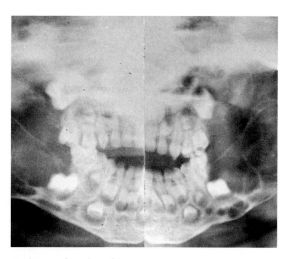

Radiograph, Cherubism

(Center) As shown in this panoramic radiograph, there are extensive bilateral multilocular radiolucencies of the posterior mandible with corresponding bone expansion. Thinning of the cortical plates is present. The normal bony architecture is lost and there is some displacement of developing teeth. Premature shedding of the deciduous dentition has been reported. Progressive enlargement has been reported to occur throughout childhood, stabilizing sometime after puberty.

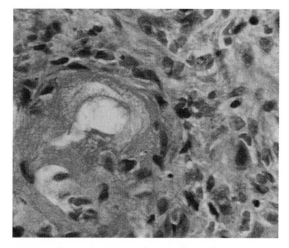

Giant Cells and Perivascular Cuffing of Cherubism   × 100

(Bottom) The microscopic features resemble those of central giant cell granuloma (see p. 98). There is no histologic similarity to fibrous dysplasia of bone. The lesions are characterized by proliferating fibroblasts in a fairly uniform pattern that produces a loose, fibrillar stroma. Giant cells with 6 to 12 nuclei each are quite plentiful. The stroma contains many small blood vessels. A distinctive peculiar eosinophilic perivascular cuffing of capillaries is sometimes observed. Special stains have revealed this material to be collagen.

PAGET'S DISEASE OF BONE

(OSTEITIS DEFORMANS)

This disease of adults, which is of unknown cause, is characterized by rapid resorption and extensive deposition of bone in a manner not related to functional needs. These two processes may go on simultaneously, or they may alternate. In the early stages resorption is more pronounced, but later osteogenesis becomes increasingly dominant, resulting in progressive enlargement of the affected bones. The newly formed bone will not stand stress; hence, if weight-bearing bones are involved, they may become compressed or bent. This is not a generalized disease of bone, although many bones may be affected. The serum calcium and phosphorus levels are usually normal; alkaline phosphatase is increased during the active phase of the disease. Sarcoma of the involved bones, arteriosclerosis, and cardiac enlargement are apt to occur in individuals with extensive Paget's disease.

(Top) Nonsymmetrical enlargement of the skull, as in this case, is often the first indication of the disease. A rib, the pelvis, the left femur, and the maxilla were also involved. Radiographic examination revealed the following: skull—"absorbent-cotton" appearance of the right parietal bone; maxilla—areas of osteoporosis adjacent to regions of sclerosis, trabeculae in other areas thin but close together, lamina dura almost completely obliterated. Hypercementosis (often present in Paget's disease of the jaws) was not evident in this case.

(Center) Marked enlargement of maxilla, with separation of the teeth. The antra were greatly diminished in size. Paget's disease affects the maxilla more frequently than the mandible.

(Bottom) The dark-blue-staining, irregularly curved cement lines indicate where resorption ceased and osteoid was again deposited. These lines appear to separate various fragments, as in a mosaic or a jigsaw puzzle. The marrow is fibrous and quite vascular. Both apposition and resorption are evident on the margins of each bone spicule. The mosaic pattern is seen only in fully developed Paget's bone.

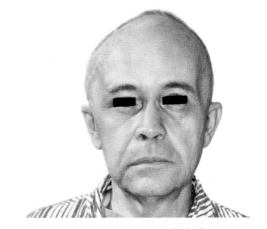

Paget's Disease, Enlargement of Skull

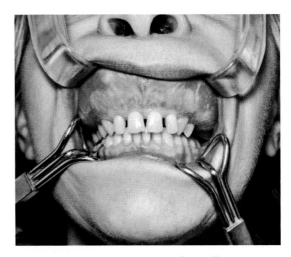

Paget's Disease, Enlargement of Maxilla

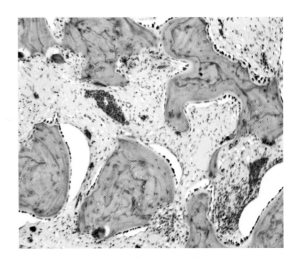

Paget's Disease, Mosaic Pattern of Bone   × 100

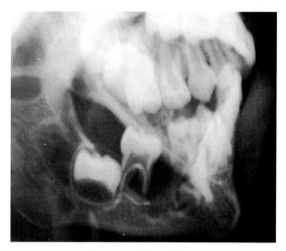

Eosinophilic Granuloma, Mandible

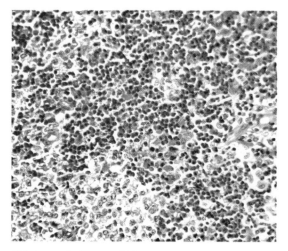

Histiocytosis-X   ×220

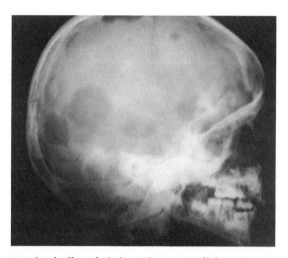

Hand-Schüller-Christian Disease, Radiolucent Areas, Skull

HISTIOCYTOSIS-X

(LANGERHANS CELL PROLIFERATION)

The term *histiocytosis* has been applied to Hand-Schüller-Christian disease (chronic disseminated histiocytosis), Letterer-Siwe disease (acute disseminated histiocytosis), and eosinophilic granuloma (local histiocytosis), indicating that these are different manifestations of a single disease process. Letterer-Siwe disease occurs in infants and rapidly involves almost all of the organs, resulting in death within a few months. Differentiation of these entities should not be based on histologic evidence alone, for the microscopic features may be quite similar.

Eosinophilic Granuloma of Bone

(Top) Osseous destruction from an eosinophilic granuloma in the mandible of a young child. this granulomatous process, which may cause pain, begins in the medullary cavity and destroys bone quite rapidly. The lesion may expand the cortex, or it may perforate it and extend into soft tissue. An eosinophilic granuloma by its manner of growth may be mistaken clinically and radiographically for a malignant neoplasm. It also may be misdiagnosed as periodontal disease. This entity, which occurs mainly in children and young adults, frequently affects only one bone. There are no extraskeletal foci or constitutional symptoms. A cure may be effected by curettement.

(Center) Biopsy specimen from the above case reveals masses of eosinophils and sheets of pale-lavender-staining vacuolated Langerhans cells typical of histiocytosis-X.

Hand-Schüller-Christian Disease

(Bottom) This 4-year-old patient had multiple radiolucent areas in the skull, as shown here, as well as exophthalmos and diabetes insipidus (Christian's triad). The two latter manifestations are due to involvement of the orbit and the pituitary gland area. In this disease there may also be a limited number of other lesions in the skin, mucous membrane, bone, and viscera.

In histiocytosis-X there is no abnormality of lipid metabolism. The proliferative cells, formerly thought to be of histiocytic origin, are now recognized as *Langerhans cells*. Langerhans cells are members of the dendritic cell system and are involved in the processing and presentation of antigen to effector cells. It is not clear whether this disease represents a neoplastic process or an exuberant reaction to some unknown stimulus.

OSTEOMYELITIS

The term *osteomyelitis* (inflammation of bone marrow) is usually reserved for a fulminating suppurative inflammatory process involving a considerable portion of a bone. In the jaws the disease may be caused by extension of a periapical infection, by entrance of organisms through wounds, or by blood-borne bacteria. Acute osteomyelitis is associated with a deep-seated, intense pain of the affected part and a rise in the patient's temperature. The inflammation, which spreads rapidly through the marrow and haversian spaces, results in the death of large amounts of bone. This bone necrosis may be in part the result of the direct effect of toxic products on the osteocytes but is caused mainly by loss of blood supply. The latter is due to thrombosis and the stripping of the periosteum from the bone by the formation of subperiosteal abscesses. Pieces of necrotic bone are separated from viable bone by osteoclastic action. These fragments of bone (sequestra), which are surrounded by pus, eventually are exfoliated. A sheath of new bone that forms at the periphery of the necrotic area is termed the *involucrum*.

(Top) Swelling of the cheek, a cutaneous abscess in the submandibular region, and a partially healed incision at the angle of the jaw are apparent. The abscess contained a fragment of necrotic bone. Several sequestra had previously been removed from an abscess that was in the region of the scar.

(Center) Extensive bone destruction in osteomyelitis of the mandible. Initially there is no radiographic evidence of this disease, for it is only after resorption or sequestration of bone has occurred that radiolucent areas can be seen. Radiographs taken after osteomyelitis has been arrested may suggest that the disease is still progressing, if the newly formed bone has not calcified completely and the necrotic bone still is being resorbed.

(Bottom) In the center of the photomicrograph is granulation tissue in which there is a small, localized collection of pus. The bone fragments are devital, for the lacunar spaces are empty. The edges of the bone are irregular, and numerous osteoclasts are lined up along the scalloped margins.

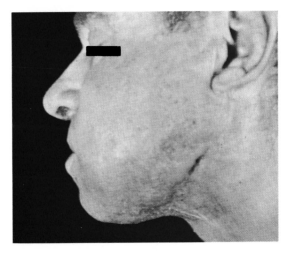

Chronic Osteomyelitis, Mandible

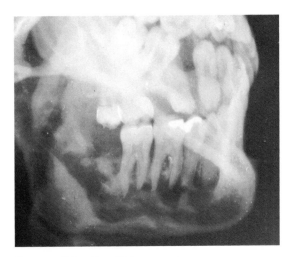

Osteomyelitis, Mandible

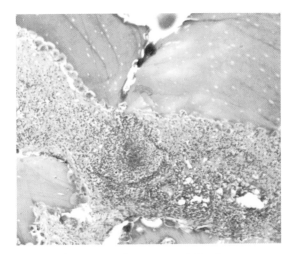

Osteomyelitis, Necrotic Bone, and Focal Suppuration × 78

VI Genetic, Metabolic, and Endocrine Disturbances

INTRODUCTION

Genetic factors are the primary causes of such disturbances as Peutz-Jegher syndrome, Gardner's syndrome, white sponge nevus, hereditary hemorrhagic telangiectasia and Mediterranean anemia, which are discussed in this chapter. Other genetic disturbances—gemination and fusion, ectodermal dysplasia, microdontia, supernumerary teeth, dentinogenesis imperfecta, amelogenesis imperfecta, dentin dysplasia, cleidocranial dysplasia, erythroblastosis fetalis, neurofibromatosis, nevoid basal cell carcinoma syndrome, and hereditary gingival fibromatosis—are discussed elsewhere in this Atlas. Genetic factors may also play an etiologic role in other diseases which are not primarily of genetic origin. Family history is most important in the diagnosis of genetic diseases. Whenever possible the members of a proband's family should be examined personally because experience has indicated that lesions which are apparent to the examining dentist may be overlooked by family members themselves. Unfortunately genetic defects cannot be "reversed" but counseling may be of great value in alleviating fears and in guiding the family toward genetic testing.

Metabolic disturbances, including melanin pigmentations, nevi, and acromegaly are among a broad group of metabolic diseases which have extraoral as well as local effects. Except for excision of oral lesions such as nevi, treatment usually falls within the responsibility of the medical profession. Nevi are more accurately classified as hamartomas, rather than benign neoplasms. Nevi may evolve into melanomas or be similar in clinical appearance to these malignancies. For this reason microscopic examination is necessary.

Endocrine disbalances result in generalized disturbances which may be reflected in the maxillofacial regions. Among these are hyperparathyroidism (osteitis fibrosa cystica), which may result in radiolucencies; acromegaly, which produces enlargement of the maxilla; and Addison's disease, which may lead to pigmentation of the oral mucosa. Agranulocytosis may be primary or result from hematopoietic depression caused by radiation or certain drugs which affect the production of leukocytes. The oral lesions may appear initially as aphthae. If these do not heal within normal periods, as with all oral lesions not definitively identified, further investigation is imperative. In these cases complete blood counts are indicated.

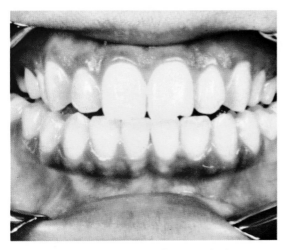

Physiologic Pigmentation (Melanosis Gingivae)

MUCOSAL MELANIN PIGMENTATION

(Top) Melanin pigmentation of the oral mucosa not associated with pathologic changes is usually termed *physiologic pigmentation.* It may occur in individuals of any racial or national origin, being seen occasionally in light-skinned people and commonly in those having darker complexions. Physiologic pigmentation is observed most often on the labial and buccal aspects of the gingiva (melanosis gingivae). Other areas involved, in order of frequency, are the buccal mucosa, hard palate, tongue, lips, and soft palate.

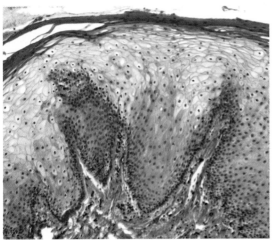

Melanosis, Mucous Membrane   × 100

(Center) This section of tissue was taken from a pigmented area in the oral mucosa. Careful examination of the basal epithelial cells will reveal that they contain a brownish-staining material, melanin, which is not ordinarily apparent in routine histologic sections of oral mucous membrane. In very heavily pigmented areas the melanin, which is formed in special cells in the basal layer (melanocytes), would be seen not only in basal epithelial cells but also in the prickle cells and in phagocytes in the lamina propria. Pigmentary changes sometimes occur in mucous membrane as well as skin following inflammatory reactions. This photomicrograph is of such a case, but the histologic findings in Addison's disease, physiologic pigmentation, or Peutz-Jeghers syndrome would be similar.

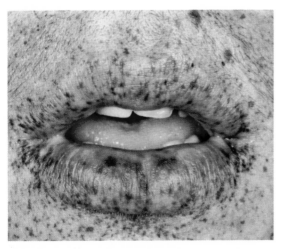

Melanin Pigmentation Associated with Intestinal Polyposis

PEUTZ-JEGHERS SYNDROME

(Bottom) Excessive melanin pigmentation in and about the oral cavity may be associated with a generalized intestinal polyposis. This relatively rare combination of findings, Peutz-Jeghers syndrome, has been observed most frequently in dark-skinned individuals and appears to be inherited. The melanin spots in this syndrome are most evident on the lips and buccal mucosa but may be present in other portions of the oral cavity, on the face (especially about the mouth), and on the digits. The patient shown, a 21-year-old Mexican, had had 2 operations for removal of intestinal polyps. Circumoral pigmentation was first noted at the age of 2. The spots became more numerous as the patient grew older.

ADDISON'S DISEASE

(Top) Hyperpigmentation of the buccal mucosa in Addison's disease (primary adrenal insufficiency). The pigmentation is due to melanin and results from lack of adrenal cortical control over pituitary secretion of melanocyte-stimulating hormone (MSH). The skin may have a bronze appearance not unlike that of dark-skinned individuals or pigmentation may be heavier in skin folds.

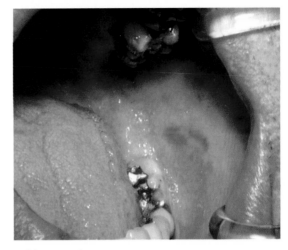

Addison's Disease

PIGMENTED NEVUS

(Center) Pigmented nevi do occur in the oral cavity but less commonly than on the skin. The hard and soft palate and the buccal and labial mucosa are the most frequently reported locations. The intramucosal (intradermal) is the commonest histologic type. It consists of aggregates of melanocytes containing varying amounts of melanin, which accounts for the clinical appearance. Differential diagnosis includes amalgam tattoo and vascular phenomena. Because it is not possible to exclude early malignant melanoma by clinical examination alone, surgical removal and pathologic examination is usually recommended (see p. 179).

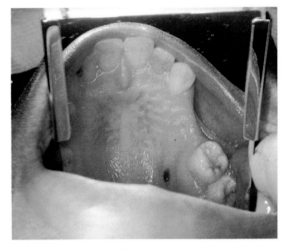

Pigmented Nevus, Palate

(Bottom) Photomicrograph of intramucosal nevus. Pigment-producing cells (melanocytes) are separated from the oral epithelium by connective tissue. Histology can be compared with that of malignant melanoma (see p. 179). The aggregates of melanocytes do not represent a true neoplasm; the more appropriate term is *hamartoma*.

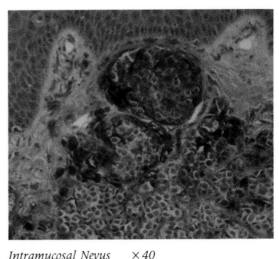

Intramucosal Nevus   ×40

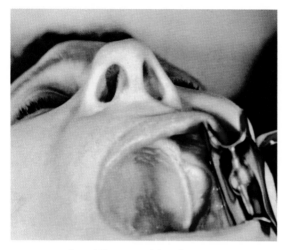

Hyperparathyroidism, Osteitis Fibrosa Cystica

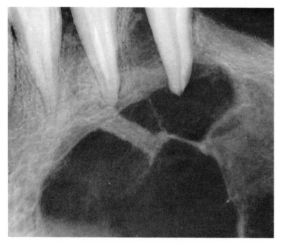

Hyperparathyroidism, Large Area of Bone Destruction and Loss of Lamina Dura

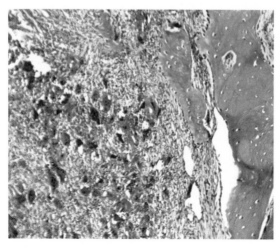

Hyperparathyroidism, Central Giant Cell Lesion   × 80

PRIMARY HYPERPARATHYROIDISM

This disease is due to an increased production of the parathyroid hormone, usually resulting from a functioning adenoma. The hormone (which regulates the renal excretion of phosphorus), when in excess, causes an immediate increase of phosphorus in the urine. This results in a fall of the serum phosphorus level. As a consequence the serum calcium rises, which in turn leads to an increased excretion of calcium in the urine. Hyperparathyroidism is therefore characterized by hypercalcemia, hypercalciuria, hypophosphatemia, and hyperphosphaturia. The most common complication of this disease is the formation of urinary calculi due to the high concentration of phosphorus and calcium in the urine. The most serious complication is the deposition of calcium in the kidney tubules (calcinosis), resulting in impaired renal function. The hypercalcemia is associated with a decrease in neuromuscular excitability which is manifested clinically by a generalized muscular weakness and constipation.

(Top)   If the calcium excretion exceeds the intake, calcium is removed from bone. In advanced cases (von Recklinghausen's disease, osteitis fibrosa cystica) large regions of bone are replaced by connective tissue containing giant cells. In the case illustrated the cortex is expanded over 2 such giant cell lesions, one in the maxilla and one on the forehead.

(Center)   The radiograph shown reveals a large region of radiolucency, resembling a cyst, traversed by a broad trabecula. The lamina dura (alveolar bone) is missing about the teeth, which resist resorption, and a smaller radiolucent lesion is adjacent to the 2nd premolar. Subperiosteal resorption along the margins of the middle phalanges and "cystic" lesions in the phalanges and long bones, as well as changes shown here in the jaws, are characteristic of osteitis fibrosa cystica.

(Bottom)   Photomicrograph of a lesion removed from a patient with this disease. This lesion is called a *brown tumor* because of its gross appearance. The color is due to numerous hemosiderin-containing macrophages and extravascular red blood cells. The stroma contains many multinucleated giant cells, similar to those found in central giant cell granuloma (see p. 98) and in cherubism (see p. 128).

ACROMEGALY

This disease of adults is caused by an overproduction of the growth hormone as a result of a functioning eosinophilic adenoma of the anterior lobe of the pituitary. Hyperfunction of eosinophilic cells occurring in young individuals (before epiphyses have closed) results in pituitary gigantism. Acromegaly is characterized by an enlargement of the nose, ears, lips, tongue, mandible, hands, and feet. It occurs with equal frequency in both sexes, and clinical manifestations usually first become apparent in the 3rd decade. In acromegaly numerous other glands of internal secretion often are indirectly involved. There may be a hyperplasia of the thymus, parathyroid, thyroid, and adrenal glands, and an atrophy of the ovaries or testes and the endocrine portion of the pancreas. Therefore, signs and symptoms related to multiple endocrine dysfunction may be associated with acromegaly. Headaches and impaired vision may result from enlargement of the adenoma.

(Top) A 65-year-old edentulous patient in whom the typical acromegalic characteristics (enlarged hands, lower jaw, and lip) first became apparent 30 years previously. In physiologic-rest position the lower anterior alveolar ridge was 1 1/2 in forward of the maxillary ridge. This fact, plus a marked macroglossia, made construction of satisfactory dentures most difficult.

(Center) Another patient, in whom separation of the teeth was the first observed clinical manifestation of acromegaly. During the active growth period of this disease the correction of occlusion, the reconstruction of partial and full dentures, and the remaking of fixed bridges are continuing problems.

HEREDITARY HEMORRHAGIC TELANGIECTASIA

(OSLER-RENDU-WEBER DISEASE)

(Bottom) This familial disease, which affects both sexes equally, is characterized by numerous dilated capillaries and venules in the skin and mucous membranes. The telangiectases may occur anywhere but generally are limited to the face, nasal mucosa, lips, tongue, floor of mouth, cheek, gastrointestinal tract, and fingertips. They may be present in childhood but usually become more numerous and noticeable in the 3rd and 4th decades. The dilated vascular spaces appear clinically as red areas, often raised. Their vascular nature is apparent when they are compressed by a glass slide, for they can be seen to fade. They are usually small, as in the case

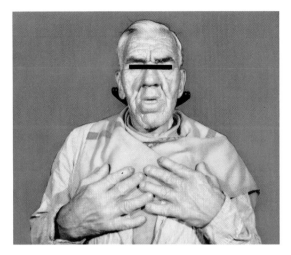

Acromegaly

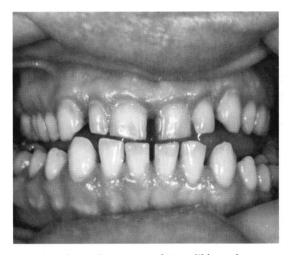

Acromegaly, Enlargement of Mandible and Separation of Teeth

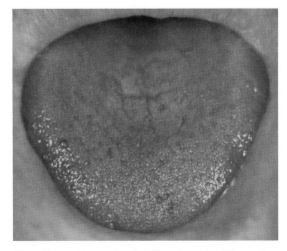

Hereditary Hemorrhagic Telangiectasia, Lingual Lesions

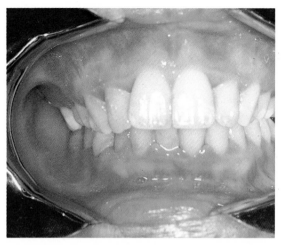

Mediterranean Anemia, Enlarged Maxilla

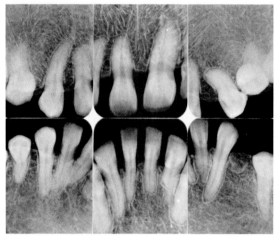

Mediterranean Anemia, Altered Bone Trabecular Pattern

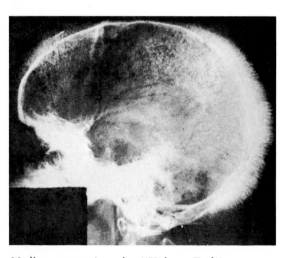

Mediterranean Anemia, "Hair-on-End" Trabeculae

HEREDITARY HEMORRHAGIC TELANGIECTASIA *(continued)*

pictured, but occasionally telangiectatic lesions as large as 0.5 cm in diameter are seen. Epistaxis is a common symptom, but bleeding may occur from any of the lesions, arising spontaneously or as a result of minor trauma. Bleeding and coagulation time, clot retraction, and platelet count are normal.

ERYTHROBLASTIC ANEMIA

(COOLEY'S ANEMIA, MEDITERRANEAN ANEMIA, THALASSEMIA)

This inherited disorder of defective hemoglobin synthesis, which may be fatal, occurs mainly in people of Mediterranean ancestry. Laboratory findings are moderately low red cell count, hypochromia, microcytosis, anisocytosis, poikilocytosis, target cells, normoblasts. There may be icterus, splenomegaly, a mongoloid facies, and a "hair-on-end" arrangement of the trabecular bone near the surface of the skull. The heterozygous form of thalassemia usually is asymptomatic but target cells (leptocytes) may appear in the blood.

(Top) In thalassemia major, a majority of patients have maxillary prominence, as is seen in this 18-year-old woman.

(Center) Dental radiographs show enlarged marrow spaces and fine trabeculae producing a hairlike pattern. This is the result of hyperplasia of the bone marrow compensating for the shortened lifespan of the erythrocytes.

(Bottom) In some individuals, a lateral skull radiograph will show elongated vertical trabeculae, producing a "hair-on-end" effect. This pattern reflects an increase in the cancellous spaces to allow for more hematopoeitic marrow.

AGRANULOCYTOSIS

(Top) In agranulocytosis (malignant neutropenia) resistance to infection is very limited because of the lack of circulating neutrophils. Often there are intraoral ulcers, as shown here, with little reaction of the tissue. Drug idiosyncrasy and prolonged use of aminopyrine, chloramphenicol, gold salts, and barbiturates are reported causes. Excessive radiation to bone marrow will also cause repression of leukocyte formation. To prevent overwhelming infection and tissue destruction, the cause should be removed and antibiotics administered until leukopoietic centers recover. Noma and death of the patient may occur without adequate treatment.

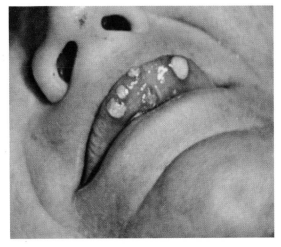

Agranulocytosis

WHITE SPONGE NEVUS

(Center) This disease, an autosomal dominant condition also is referred to as congenital keratosis and as familial white folded gingivostomatosis. It is characterized by extensive thick, keratinized lesions in the oral mucosa. The keratinized areas have a shiny, opalescent surface, which may be pebbly or filamentous in character. The lesions are soft and spongy and often are traversed by numerous deep grooves. Occasionally small vesicles are seen. The entire oral mucosa, as well as other mucous membranes, may be involved. This harmless disease should be distinguished from other keratotic oral lesions of more serious character. The diagnosis should be based on familial history, clinical appearance, and histologic findings.

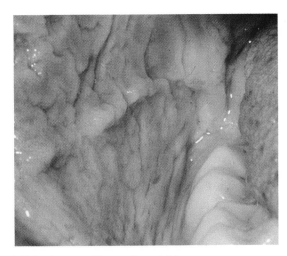

White Sponge Nevus, Buccal Mucosa

(Bottom) The histologic findings are distinctive and diagnostic. The epithelium is thickened, and the rete pegs are broad and fused. Parakeratin is present in varying amounts on the surface and, in some regions, extends deeply to the basal layer. A marked edema, both intracellular and extracellular, is evident in the prickle cell layer. Small vesicles are occasionally formed. Several of the prickle cells are devoid of nuclei and cytoplasm; others have small amounts of red cytoplasm around nuclei; and in others the nuclei are of normal size and dense red cytoplasm fills the cells. The detailed cellular changes cannot be seen at this magnification.

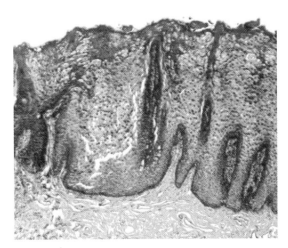

White Sponge Nevus, Biopsy Specimen from Above Case × 40

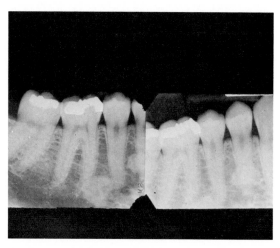

Gardner's Syndrome, Multiple Osteomas

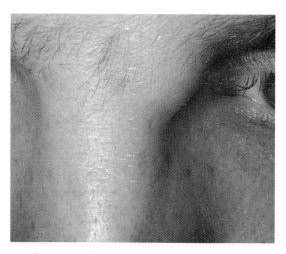

Gardner's Syndrome, Sebaceous Cyst

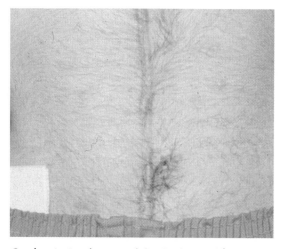

Gardner's Syndrome, Abdominal Scar from Colonic Resection

GARDNER'S SYNDROME

Gardner's syndrome is an autosomal dominant genetic condition that shows frequent involvement of the teeth and jaw bones. Supernumerary teeth and multiple osteomas are rather constant findings in patients with the syndrome. Osteomas central in bone are characteristic. When osteomas are located peripherally they may be palpated on physical examination.

(Top) The occurrence of osteomas in the jaws, skull, and long bones is one of the components of the syndrome. These periapical radiographs are of a 22-year-old male and show multiple osteomas. The patient reported that supernumerary teeth had been removed several years earlier.

(Center) Other components of the syndrome include sebaceous cysts and fibrous tumors. The most serious manifestation of the syndrome is colorectal adenocarcinoma. The photograph shows a sebaceous cyst on this same 22-year-old male.

(Bottom) Abdominal scar from colonic resection in the same patient. Persons with the syndrome are at 12 times greater risk for developing colorectal cancer. Typical symptoms include rectal bleeding, diarrhea, and abdominal pain. Detection of elevated serum levels of ornithine decarboxylase (ODC) can result in earlier identification of patients at risk, before colorectal cancer develops. Patients with Gardner's syndrome should be referred to gastroenterologists as soon as the syndrome is recognized.

LOSS OF TONGUE PAPILLAE

(BALD TONGUE; ATROPHIC GLOSSITIS)

Absence or loss of filiform papillae from the tongue has been reported to be associated with vitamin B complex malnutrition (especially riboflavin deficiency), pernicious anemia, Plummer-Vinson syndrome, candidosis, and increasing age. The clinical appearance of a bald tongue is in itself not diagnostic but only suggestive of a particular disease.

(Top) The fungiform papillae on the anterior portion of the tongue are enlarged. Bilateral angular cheilosis and an increase in the vertical markings on the left side of the upper lip are also apparent. The prominence of the fungiform papillae, a very early tongue change in vitamin B deficiency, is often overlooked. In this case the malnutrition was dietary, and there was a quick response to oral administration of vitamin B complex.

(Center) This patient suffers from pernicious anemia, a disease due to lack of an intrinsic factor in the gastric secretion without which absorption of the erythrocyte-maturing factor (vitamin B_{12}) is impaired. Laboratory findings are very low red cell count, macrocytosis, poikilocytosis, anisocytosis, normochromia, hypersegmented neutrophils, numerous megaloblasts in bone marrow, achlorhydria. Various signs and symptoms related to changes in hematologic, gastrointestinal, and neurologic systems may be present. Among these are greenish-yellow skin color and glossitis, as shown in the illustration. The dorsal surface of the tongue is atrophic, and the margins are red. In other cases the tongue may be painful, and the lateral margins and tip fiery red.

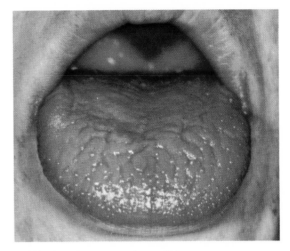

Mild Vitamin B Complex Deficiency

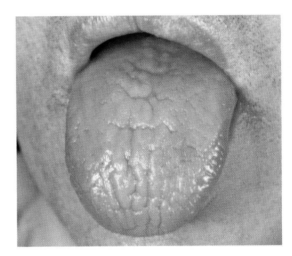

Pernicious Anemia, Atrophic Glossitis

ANGULAR CHEILOSIS

(Bottom) Angular cheilosis in vitamin B complex deficiency. The lesion, which extends horizontally, involves both mucous membrane and skin. This patient was on an improperly balanced diet consisting chiefly of rice. Angular cheilosis may also result from a decrease in the vertical dimension, from licking the corners of the mouth (perlèche), or from candidiasis. With a marked loss of the vertical dimension, deep folds that slant downward are produced at the corners of the mouth. These become macerated because they are constantly bathed in saliva. It is not uncommon to find that a patient has angular cheilosis from both loss of vertical dimension and vitamin B complex deficiency.

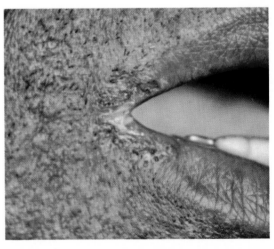

Vitamin B Complex Deficiency, Angular Cheilosis

INTRODUCTION

Neoplasms are autonomous new growths. They arise spontaneously, and their growth is not limited by the biologic restraints that control the growth of other cells. Usually they are nonfunctional, but when functional they are independent of biologic controls. They always produce deleterious effects and may cause the death of the host.

Neoplasms may be classified in several ways. They are divided into benign and malignant types. Malignant neoplasms are those that have the potential to kill the host unless they are eliminated by surgery, radiation therapy, chemotherapy, or combined treatment. Rarely they may regress without therapy. They are anaplastic, invade surrounding tissue, and may metastasize by lymph or blood vessels. The individual cells exhibit variations in size and shape, hyperchromatism, abnormal mitotic figures, altered polarity, and variations in the proportions of nuclear material. Malignant epithelial neoplasms are termed *carcinomas,* and those of mesenchymal tissues are termed *sarcomas.* *Melanomas* are malignant tumors of melanocytes; malignant tumors of lymphoid tissues are termed *malignant lymphomas.*

Benign neoplasms grow slowly and remain localized. They closely resemble the cells from which they were derived. Benign neoplasms of stratified squamous epithelium are termed *papillomas* and those of glandular epithelium are *adenomas.* The terms for most neoplasms of supporting structures are derived by adding the suffix "oma" to the histologic designation of the tissue or cells of origin, hence *fibroma, osteoma, chondroma, lipoma.*

The term *tumor* originally meant a swelling but now is used generally and loosely as a synonym for neoplasm. The aforementioned characteristics of benign and malignant neoplasms are applicable in a general manner, but it is essential to have specific knowledge about each entity. Histologic appearances do not necessarily reflect the potential clinical behavior or course of a given neoplasm. Each neoplasm should be studied thoroughly and each type considered as a different disease.

Neoplasia is related to the inherent ability of cells to multiply. In normal growth, in hyperplasia, and in repair there is a regulating factor that probably is coded into the DNA. When this inhibitory factor is diminished (e.g., in AIDS [see p. 121]) or when the stimulation for growth is too great, a neoplasm may result. Once transformation to a neoplastic cell has occurred the trait of uncontrolled growth is transmitted to successive generations of cells. Intrinsic factors appear to condition cells for neoplastic transformation. Genetic factors are suggested in many neoplasms but are clearly apparent in only a few. Oncogenes, which are associated with neoplasia, may be involved in the initiation and progression of tumor cells in squamous cell carcinoma and other oral neoplasms.

Extrinsic factors that appear to be important in initiation of neoplasia include exposure to coal tar and its products (especially from tobacco), sunlight, ionizing radiation, chronic irritation, and viral infection.

Prevention is the ultimate goal for solving the cancer problem but at present the mortality rates can be reduced only by elimination of recognizable extrinsic factors, early diagnosis, and early treatment. Treatment of neoplasms should be done by those especially qualified but early detection is the responsibility of every practitioner. One should have a high level of suspicion, and any lesion that has existed for 2 wk should be biopsied unless its exact nature is known.

TNM Classification, 3rd Edition

DEFINITION OF TNM
Primary Tumor (T)
(Lip and Oral Cavity)

TX Primary tumor cannot be assessed
T0 No evidence of primary tumor
Tis Carcinoma *in situ*
T1 Tumor 2 cm or less in greatest dimension
T2 Tumor more than 2 cm but not more than 4 cm in greatest dimension
T3 Tumor more than 4 cm in greatest dimension
T4 (lip) Tumor invades adjacent structures (e.g., through cortical bone, tongue, skin of neck)
T4 (oral cavity) Tumor invades adjacent structures (e.g., through cortical bone into deep [extrinsic] muscle of tongue, maxillary sinus, skin)

Regional Lymph Nodes (N)
NX Regional lymph nodes cannot be assessed
N0 No regional lymph node metastasis
N1 Metastasis in a single ipsilateral lymph node, 3 cm or less in greatest dimension
N2 Metastasis in a single ipsilateral lymph node, more than 3 cm but not more than 6 cm in greatest dimension; or in multiple ipsilateral lymph nodes, none more than 6 cm in greatest dimension; or in bilateral or contralateral lymph nodes, none more than 6 cm in greatest dimension
N2a: Metastasis in single ipsilateral lymph node more than 3 cm but not more than 6 cm in greatest dimension
N2b: Metastasis in multiple ipsilateral lymph nodes, none more than 6 cm in greatest dimension
N2c: Metastasis in bilateral or contralateral lymph nodes none more than 6 cm in greatest dimension

N3 Metastasis in a lymph node more than 6 cm in greatest dimension

Distant Metastasis (M)
MX Presence of distant metastasis cannot be assessed
M0 No distant metastasis
M1 Distant metastasis

Stage Grouping

	T	N	M
Stage 0	Tis	N0	M0
Stage I	T1	N0	M0
Stage II	T2	N0	M0
Stage III	T3	N0	M0
	T1	N1	M0
	T2	N1	M0
	T3	N1	M0
Stage IV	T4	N0, N1	M0
	Any T	N2, N3	M0
	Any T	Any N	M1

Reprinted with permission of the American Joint Committee on Cancer

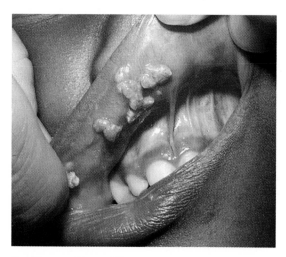

Papillomas, Upper Lip

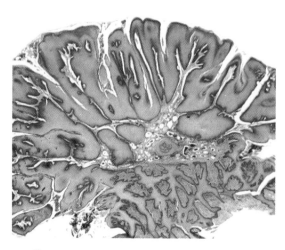

Papilloma, Lip

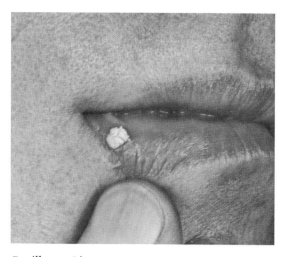

Papilloma ×6

PAPILLOMA

Papillomas are benign neoplasms of squamous epithelium. Their exophytic growth produces various clinical patterns. Papillomas may have a broad base firmly attached to the surface (sessile), or may arise from a slender stalk (pedunculated) and be freely movable. The surface of the lesion is white due to the high degree of keratinization and tendency for retention of keratin. Some papillomas consist of limp, white, threadlike projections that resemble somewhat the hyperplastic filiform papillae of hairy tongue; in others the projections are blunt, short, and stiff; and in still others the surface has a cauliflowerlike appearance. A pedunculated papilloma may be readily diagnosed clinically, but without histologic examination the sessile, cauliflower type is difficult to distinguish from a papillomatous carcinoma.

(Top) Papillomas arising from the upper lip. Papillomas are usually small in size and single, but are sometimes large and multiple as in this case. Children occasionally have numerous lesions (juvenile papillomata) in the larynx, pharynx, and oral cavity which, until the age of puberty, tend to grow rapidly and to recur if removed.

(Center) This sessile type of papilloma has the clinical appearance of a wart (verruca vulgaris). The dermal verrucca is an epithelial overgrowth which is induced by papilloma virus. The papilloma is always sessile and markedly hornified, and the rete pegs at its periphery bend in toward the center. Intranuclear inclusion bodies occasionally may be identified in verruca.

(Bottom) Photomicrograph showing how the proliferating epithelium of a papilloma protrudes outward, forming numerous folds. Each fold is supported by a thin, vascular, fibrous connective tissue core. Cell detail cannot be seen at this magnification, but it is evident that the epithelium has a uniform character and the dark-staining basal layer is intact. Human papilloma virus (HPV) can usually be identified in these lesions with special stains. Compare with papillomatous carcinoma (p. 172, *top*).

FIBROMA

A true fibroma of the oral cavity is rare. The term is often used, however, to designate localized proliferations of fibrous tissue that are hyperplasias resulting from long-standing irritation. Such non-neoplastic fibrous lesions are found in the buccal mucosa opposite the occlusal line, the lateral border of the tongue, the vestibular mucosa, and the lip. They may be either sessile or pedunculated and are usually smooth-surfaced, firm, and asymptomatic. These fibrous nodules are comparable with the hyperplasias from denture irritation (see p. 94). Rather than implying neoplasia by describing such lesions as fibromas, it is more accurate to designate them as areas of subepithelial fibrosis, or as fibrous hyperplasia.

(Top) Fibrous lesions in this location are usually the result of sucking and chewing on the cheek. They continue to grow slowly as long as they are traumatized, the increase in size being related to productive inflammation. If the irritation ceases, the lesion will stop enlarging and may decrease slightly in size. Histologic examination of this so-called fibroma in the buccal mucosa revealed compressed stratified squamous epithelium covering a core of dense, hyalinized fibrous connective tissue.

(Center) The central portion of this sessile lesion is composed of dense fibrous connective tissue. The covering epithelium is somewhat thinned but intact.

(Bottom) A section from a continuously enlarging growth in the floor of the mouth. This is a true fibroma. There is a marked fibroblastic proliferation. The intensity of nuclear staining is uniform, and the nuclei vary little in size and shape. (Compare this lesion with its malignant counterpart, p. 178.)

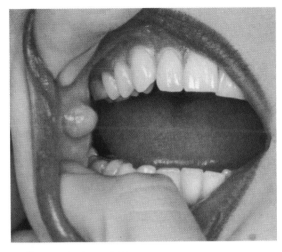

"Fibroma," Buccal Mucosa

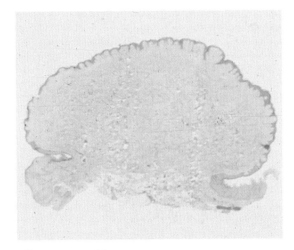

Fibroma   ×10

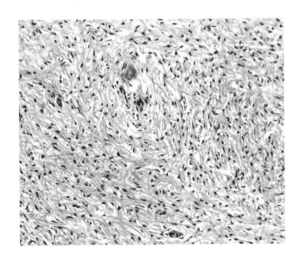

Fibroma   ×100

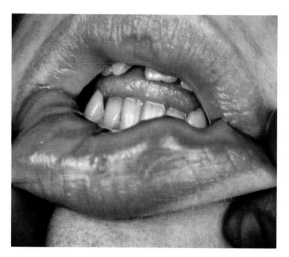

Lipoma, Lip

LIPOMA

(Top)   A lipoma consists of adult fat cells that are grouped into lobules by vascular fibrous connective tissue septae. This type of neoplasm usually appears clinically as a light-yellow spherical enlargement that is soft to palpation. In the case illustrated the lesion is deeply situated, and therefore the characteristic yellow color is not apparent on the surface. Lipomas are common in the subcutaneous tissue of the trunk, upper extremities, and neck, but are less frequently encountered in the oral cavity. The most common locations in the oral regions are the buccal mucosa and the floor of the mouth. Lipomas grow slowly, and malignant transformation is rare.

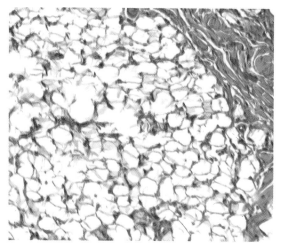

Lipoma   × 100

(Center)   Supporting stroma is apparent at upper right. The clear circular structures are fat cells; those cut in the plane of their nuclei (which are compressed against the cell membrane) resemble signet rings. The lipid present is typical of that found in normal fat and is dissolved away in preparation, but may be demonstrated by special staining of frozen sections. It is generally believed that the fat in a lipoma is not available for nutritional purposes. Many fatty tumors contain fibrous connective tissue in excess of the usual quantity of supporting stroma in adipose tissue. These are termed *fibrolipomas*.

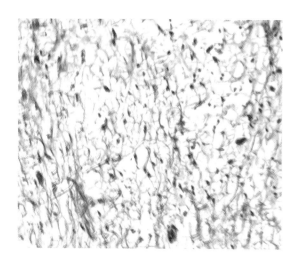

Myxoma   × 100

MYXOMA

(Bottom)   Myxomas are benign neoplasms representative of the embryonal stroma. They are composed of scattered stellate cells having delicate processes widely separated by mucoid material. Although benign, they are locally aggressive, nonencapsulated infiltrating lesions. They occur in the soft tissues of extremities, and in joints and periarticular structures, sometimes producing marked destruction of joints. They seldom occur within bone. True myxomas are rare in the jaws, but some arise from the dental papilla. Although they have a similar histologic pattern, these odontogenic myxomas do not exhibit the aggressive behavior of the nonodontogenic myxomas, and cure may be accomplished by less radical surgery. The lesion in the jaw often is lobulated and radiographically may simulate the ameloblastoma (see p. 155).

OSTEOMA

The osteoma is composed almost entirely of well-differentiated mature bone. Although not so common as tori, osteomas occasionally arise in the jaws. They may be peripheral or central. Skeletal neoplasms arising from marrow, vessels, or nerves usually are not considered to be of osseous origin.

(Top) Osteoma of moderate size on the lateral border of mandible near the premolar region. The mucosa overlying this hard, bony enlargement is thin and blanched. Peripheral osseous nodules arise from the periosteum, whereas central tumors arise from the endosteum. They increase in size slowly and generally are asymptomatic. Osteomas that are central in origin may cause some expansion of the cortical plates but do not produce the type of nodular mass seen here. It sometimes is difficult to differentiate between peripheral osteomas and hyperplasias of bone (exostoses) other than those commonly designated as tori (see p. 23.) Generally the osteoma exhibits a greater capacity for growth and contains immature bone, while hyperostoses show laminated growth and mature compact bone.

(Center) Radiograph of the osteoma shown in the preceding picture. The sharply defined area of increased density can be observed superimposed over the 1st molar and 2nd premolar. The degree of radiopacity of the lesion indicates that the osseous structure is compact.

(Bottom) In this section of a dense osteoma of the type shown above, numerous heavy, irregular trabeculae are apparent. These are separated by small spaces containing vascular fibrous connective tissue. In older lesions fibrous connective tissue is nearly absent, while it is more plentiful in younger ones.

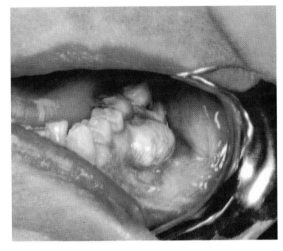

Peripheral Osteoma

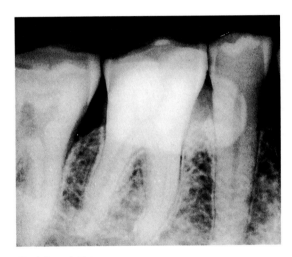

Peripheral Osteoma

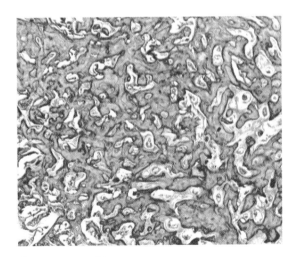

Osteoma   × 14

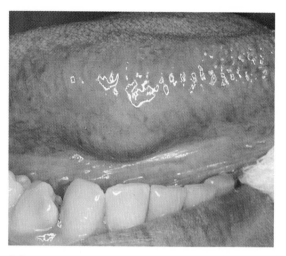

Schwannoma, Tongue

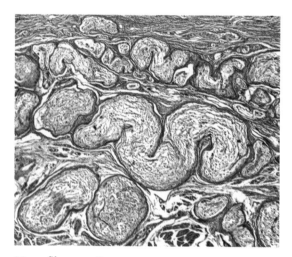

Neurofibroma, Tongue   × 70

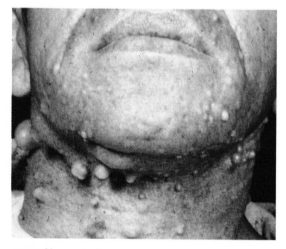

Neurofibromatosis

SCHWANNOMA

(NEURILEMOMA)

(Top)   A Schwannoma is a neoplastic overgrowth of Schwann cells, which normally constitute the neurilemmal sheath of a peripheral nerve (see p. 8). These benign tumors usually are small, asymptomatic, well circumscribed, and grow slowly. Schwannomas are fairly common neoplasms. They are seldom painful. Histologically, they consist of Schwann cells with some palisaded nuclei adjacent to hyaline areas (Verocay bodies).

NEUROFIBROMA

The neurofibroma is characterized by an overgrowth of all the elements of a peripheral nerve. These tissues (axon cylinders, Schwann cells, and fibrous connective tissue) may be arranged in a variety of patterns in different lesions. Neurofibromas occur singly but often are multiple and constitute the main feature of neurofibromatosis (von Recklinghausen's disease of skin). In this disease, which follows a genetic pattern, there may also be various developmental disturbances, *café au lait* spots on the skin, and nevi occurring alone or in association with neurofibromas.

(Center)   A plexiform type of neurofibroma with proliferation within the nerve sheath, causing swollen, tortuous nerve fasciculi. The specimen was removed from the tongue of a 6-year-old boy because that organ was so large that it interfered with mastication, swallowing, and enunciation. The patient probably suffered from multiple endocrine neoplasia syndrome (Sipple's syndrome).

(Bottom)   Numerous cutaneous neurofibromas that had been present for several years. There is a slight tendency for neurofibromas to undergo sarcomatous change. However, it is generally agreed that once the diagnosis has been established by biopsy, further surgical procedures are undesirable unless there is clinical suspicion of malignant transformation.

GRANULAR CELL TUMOR

(MYOBLASTOMA)

(Top) Granular cell tumor (myoblastic myoma, granular cell myoblastoma) is a benign neoplasm consisting of large polyhedral cells with abundant granular cytoplasm. Electron microscope studies indicate the histogenesis may be of neural (Schwann cell) origin and that more than one type of cell may be the progenitor. They do not appear to rise from skeletal muscle cells. Myoblastomas occur in sites other than skeletal muscle. They are most frequently found in the tongue, but may occur in the lip or gingiva. Only rarely does a patient have more than a single lesion, or one that exceeds 2 cm in diameter. Pseudoepitheliomatous hyperplasia may be associated with some myoblastomas. The gingival lesion when present at birth may be termed *congenital epulis of the newborn.* Electron microscopic studies suggest that the congenital epulis type originates from mesenchymal cells and is a reactive lesion.

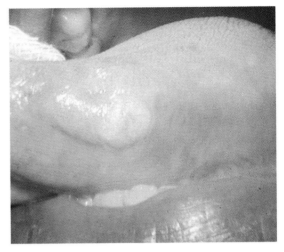

Granular Cell Tumor, Tongue

(Center) In this low-power view of a granular cell tumor of the tongue, the neoplastic cells are confined to a triangular area which stains a light purple. The covering epithelium, devoid of papillae, appears clinically as a smooth red lesion. The long, narrow, reddish-staining strips of tissue in intimate relation to the neoplasm are skeletal muscle fibers.

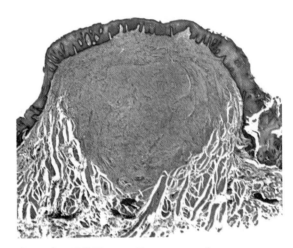

Granular Cell Tumor, Tongue ×6

(Bottom) This photomicrograph suggests early invasive carcinoma in the region overlying a granular cell tumor, but the changes are typical of intense *pseudoepitheliomatous hyperplasia* stimulated by the underlying cells. Misinterpretation of the epithelial changes may result in unnecessary radical surgery.

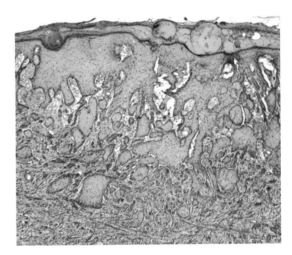

Pseudoepitheliomatous Hyperplasia Over Granular Cell Tumor ×10

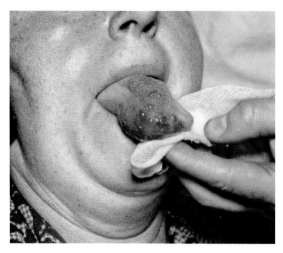

Hemangioma, Tongue

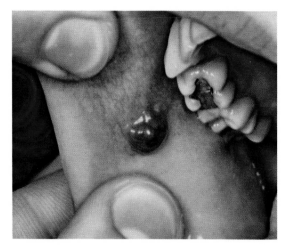

Hemangioma, Buccal Mucosa

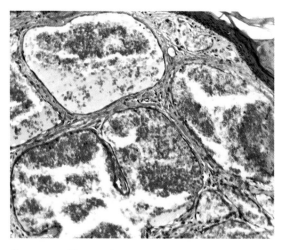

Cavernous Hemangioma   ×40

HEMANGIOMA

Hemangiomas are benign tumors of blood vessels. They occur most frequently in the skin of the face and neck but are not rare in the tongue, buccal mucosa, and lip. The bone, viscera, and central nervous system may be involved. The majority of skin lesions are present at birth and remain static. Some of the congenital lesions are considered developmental anomalies, not neoplasms. Varicosities and trauma-induced arteriovenous aneurysms (traumatic angioma) may show similar patterns. Histologically, hemangiomas may be divided into two types: capillary and cavernous.

(Top)   Large cavernous hemangioma that had been present on the tongue since birth. Hemangiomas and lymphangiomas are the most common causes of macroglossia. Occasionally the whole tongue is involved and enlarges to such a size that it cannot be retained in the oral cavity (see p. 25).

(Center)   Slightly lobulated hemangioma in the buccal mucosa. Hemangiomas are blue, purple, or purplish-red in color and usually blanch when pressure is applied. Except for the port-wine stains, most of these lesions are elevated.

(Bottom)   At the upper right-hand corner of the photomicrograph is a portion of the covering epithelium, which is stretched. In the underlying connective tissue there are several large, thin-walled, endothelial-lined spaces containing numerous red blood cells. This lesion is classified as a cavernous hemangioma because the vascular spaces are of a large size. It is generally believed that these spaces intercommunicate. Hemangiomas are not encapsulated.

Hemangiomas may extend into the maxillary or mandibular bone, producing a soap-bubble–like appearance radiographically. Angiography is useful in demonstrating the location, extent, and blood supply of hemangiomas.

STURGE-WEBER SYNDROME

(Top) Encephalotrigeminal angiomatosis (Sturge–Weber syndrome) is a syndrome complex that includes hemangiomas of the skin that follow the distribution of the trigeminal nerve (flaming nevus) leptomeningeal angiomas, intracranial calcifications, contralateral hemiplegia, and epilepsy. The syndrome should be differentiated from uncomplicated flaming nevus of the face (port-wine stain), which is not associated with the other symptoms.

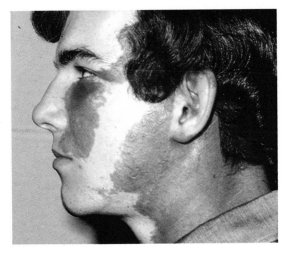

Flaming Nevus of Sturge–Weber Syndrome

LYMPHANGIOMA

Lymphangiomas are composed of numerous lymph vessels, and most of them—like hemangiomas—are not true neoplasms. One form of this lesion, cystic hygroma, has already been discussed on page 19. Lymphangiomas are not so common as hemangiomas. If they contain small lymph spaces they are termed *lymphangioma simplex;* if the spaces are large, the lesion is designated as *cystic lymphangioma.* When lymphangiomas are very superficial, small lymph-filled vesicles may erupt on the surface.

(Center) Marked enlargement of the upper lip from a large lymphangioma. This lesion, which was present at birth, remained static for several years. Lymphangiomas are most frequently encountered in the tongue, lips, neck, and inguinal regions. Clinically, the color of the skin overlying a lymphangioma is normal or slightly brownish.

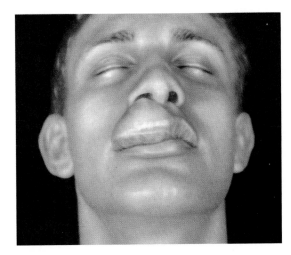

Lymphangioma, Lip

(Bottom) This is a section from a tongue that was markedly enlarged from a cystic lymphangioma. In three areas there are lakes of homogeneous light-lavender-staining material, which is lymph. This material is contained in channels that are lined by a few flattened endothelial cells. In some instances macroglossia results from both hemangiomatous and lymphangiomatous elements. Histologically, a lymphangioma may be distinguished from a hemangioma only by the absence of red blood cells in the endothelium-lined spaces. If the tissue is fixed in alcohol, this criterion cannot be used.

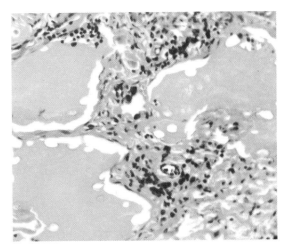

Lymphangioma   × 100

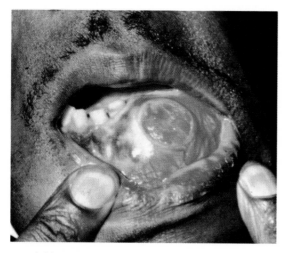

Ameloblastoma, Mandible

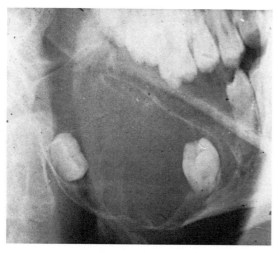

Ameloblastoma, Mandible

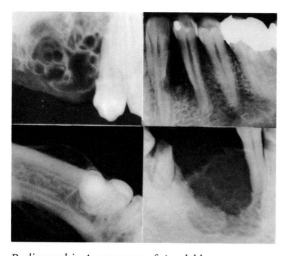

Radiographic Appearance of Ameloblastoma, Four Cases

NEOPLASMS OF ODONTOGENIC ORIGIN

Three fundamental types of neoplasm arise from odontogenic tissue or from cells with a potential for forming dental tissues. They may be purely epithelial (ameloblastomas), purely mesenchymal (odontogenic myxomas; fibromas), or mixtures of epithelial and mesenchymal elements in varying proportions (mixed odontogenic tumors). The last are identified by combinations of terms reflecting their histologic character, such as compound and complex odontomas, ameloblastic fibroma, ameloblastic fibro-odontoma.

(Top) Large mandibular ameloblastoma of 6 years duration which had been inadequately removed 4 years earlier. Ameloblastomas usually are unicentric, nonfunctional, intermittent in growth, anatomically benign, and clinically persistent. They are five times more frequent in the mandible than in the maxilla and most commonly are discovered during the 4th decade of life. Although metastasis is extremely rare, ameloblastomas and other odontogenic neoplasms may undergo malignant change. Ameloblastomas found in the lung are not necessarily metastatic; they may result from aspiration of neoplastic cells during surgical removal of an oral tumor or may represent primary adenocarcinomas with histology similar to ameloblastoma.

(Center) Radiograph of a large mandibular ameloblastoma which extends from the premolar region into the ramus. The lobulated neoplasm has expanded the cortex and displaced the adjacent teeth. Extensions of the ameloblastoma into medullary bone spaces may resemble proliferations of the dental lamina and result in recurrences if the tumor is not completely enucleated or resected.

(Bottom) Small areas of bone destruction from ameloblastomas such as might be revealed by routine radiographic examination preceding clinical suspicion of the tumor. The radiolucent area in the upper right film between the canine and the 1st premolar might be confused with a periodontal pocket. The occlusal view shows expansion of the cortex without perforation, which is typical, even in large lesions. Radiographic findings are not pathognomonic for ameloblastomas. Histologic examinations are required for definitive diagnosis. Ameloblastomas may vary greatly in histologic pattern, but in each instance the tumor includes cells that resemble those seen in the enamel organ. Some of the component cells are often so arranged as to simulate structures seen in some early stage of tooth development. These neoplasms may be solid or cystic, but this is not a pertinent division, because the

solid type is probably just a young tumor. The ameloblastoma is essentially benign but locally invasive and occasionally may kill by extension to vital structures. It is a central tumor that expands but usually does not perforate the cortical plates. Ameloblastoma may arise from remnants of the dental lamina, from the periodontal debris of Malassez, and from the enamel organ. It also may arise from the lining cells of a dentigerous cyst.

(Top) In this solid type of ameloblastoma there is very little connective tissue stroma, and the numerous islands of epithelial cells closely approximate each other. These islands are bordered by palisaded columnar cells that resemble ameloblasts. In the central portion of each aggregation is a loose network of cells suggestive of stellate reticulum. Solid ameloblastomas often contain double rows of columnar cells quite like the dental lamina.

(Center) Typical pattern of ameloblastoma with epithelial islands having peripheral cells representative of ameloblasts surrounding delicate tissue of stellate reticulum type. A layer of cells suggesting stratum intermedium sometimes is present. Liquefaction, which can be responsible for the development of microcysts, is evident.

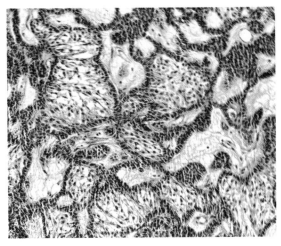

Ameloblastoma, Plexiform Pattern ×100

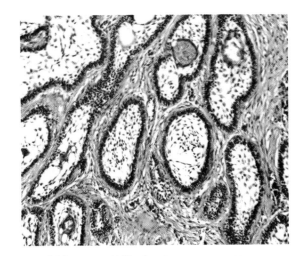

Ameloblastoma, Follicular Pattern ×100

(Bottom) At the lower right a typical ameloblastoma with microcysts is replacing bone. The three large circular areas show tumor invasion into vascular spaces. All are cystic, and that at the upper left has an area of solid tumor adjacent. The cystic spaces are lined by flat, squamatoid epithelium typical of reduced enamel epithelium. If the biopsy specimen had been small and included only cystic elements of this type, it might have been misinterpreted as an odontogenic cyst.

A unicystic (cytocystic) type of ameloblastoma has been described as being less aggressive and usually associated with a preexisting odontogenic cyst.

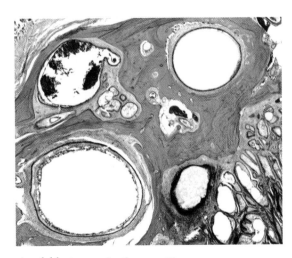

Ameloblastoma, Cystic ×15

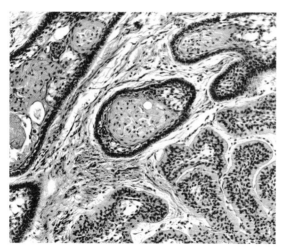

Ameloblastoma with Squamous Metaplasia × 100

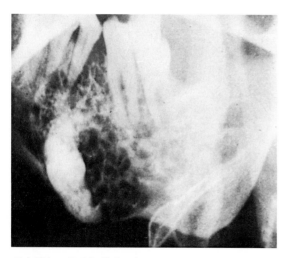

Calcifying Epithelial Odontogenic Tumor

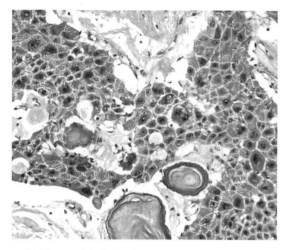

Calcifying Epithelial Odontogenic Tumor × 100

NEOPLASMS OF ODONTOGENIC ORIGIN *(continued)*

(Top) The epithelial islands in this section of ameloblastoma have columnar cells on their surfaces. In the center are elements suggestive of stellate reticulum and nests of squamatoid cells. Ameloblastomas showing squamous metaplasia are designated *acanthomatous ameloblastomas.* This variety of lesion in a very few instances has undergone malignant change.

The so-called pigmented ameloblastoma appears to be of neural crest origin and is now termed *pigmented neuroectodermal tumor of infancy.*

(Center) Radiograph demonstrating *calcifying epithelial odontogenic tumor* (Pindborg tumor) involving the mandible. Like the ameloblastoma, this tumor shows a predilection for occurrence in the mandible. There is a radiographic pattern of radiolucency and radiopacity because of the foci of mineralization in the tumor. The tumor is slow-growing and locally invasive.

(Bottom) Calcifying epithelial odontogenic tumor (Pindborg tumor) is composed of sheets of polyhedral epithelial cells in a connective tissue stroma. These closely packed cells sometimes are divided into islands or strands by the stroma. The nuclei, variable in size and shape, may be well differentiated or pleomorphic, as in this illustration. The slightly eosinophilic cytoplasm degenerates and tends to calcify, with the formation of Liesegang rings. Calcification may also occur in collagenous tissue. Amyloid has been described in the tumor cells and stroma. Most frequently this tumor is found in association with a nonerupted tooth although extraosseous lesions have been reported. Radiographically, the calcifications may cause radiopaque flecks in the radiolucent lesion.

(Top) Radiograph of *adenomatoid odontogenic tumor* showing a well-delineated radiolucency in the anterior mandible. These tumors present as unilocular radiolucencies which may contain small radiopaque foci. They have been reported associated with unerupted teeth, therefore resembling dentigerous cysts (see p. 31). Most patients are under 20 years of age.

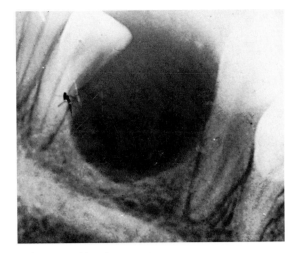

Adenomatoid Odontogenic Tumor

(Center) Several ductlike structures lined by a single row of columnar epithelial cells are apparent. Near the middle of the left and right borders are other structures typical of the *adenomatoid odontogenic tumor* (adenoameloblastoma). These structures consist of a double row of tall epithelial cells with basally placed nuclei. Between these two rows of cells is a dark-staining material that appears to have been secreted by these cells. The lesion most frequently appears as a cystlike radiolucency, associated with a nonerupted tooth in the maxillary canine region of a teenager. It grows slowly by expansion and is not aggressive. Conservative treatment is indicated; recurrences, although rare, have been reported.

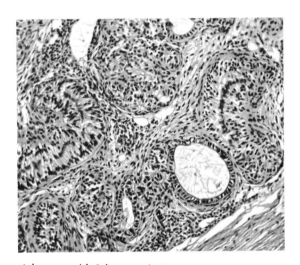

Adenomatoid Odontogenic Tumor   × 100

(Bottom) An *odontogenic myxoma* is a neoplasm of the mesenchymal portion of a tooth bud. It consists of a delicate, loosely arranged fibrous tissue containing many stellate fibroblasts. It closely simulates myxomas of soft tissues. Usually, they are painless and have a soap-bubble appearance radiographically. Since odontogenic myxomas grow progressively and do recur, excision to tumor-free margins is recommended. In this photomicrograph, the myxoma has infiltrated between bone trabeculae.

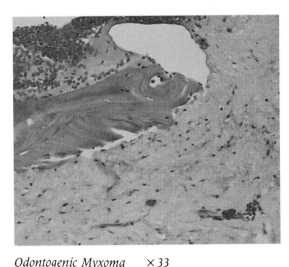

Odontogenic Myxoma   × 33

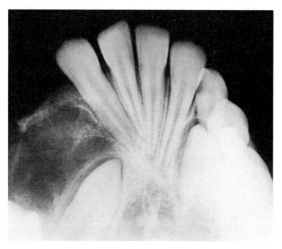

Ameloblastic Fibroma

NEOPLASMS OF
ODONTOGENIC ORIGIN *(continued)*

(Top) Radiograph of a mixed tissue odontogenic tumor, the *ameloblastic fibroma*. The appearance may be unilocular or, as in this case, multilocular. Clinically, the tumor is generally encountered in children and teenagers. It enlarges by gradual expansion. Conservative enucleation is the treatment of choice. There is little tendency for recurrence.

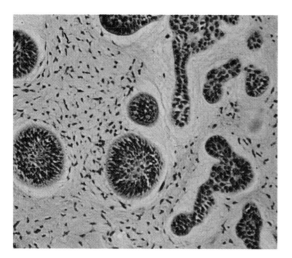

Ameloblastic Fibroma × 100

(Center) There are two neoplastic components of the ameloblastic fibroma, both arising from the tooth bud. Along the two lateral borders of the photomicrograph are portions of structures that resemble enamel organs. These constitute the epithelial portion of the neoplasm. The rest of the tissue is proliferating fibrous connective tissue that resembles dental pulp tissue. The proportion of fibrous and epithelial tissue varies from one tumor to another, as does the cellularity of the stroma.

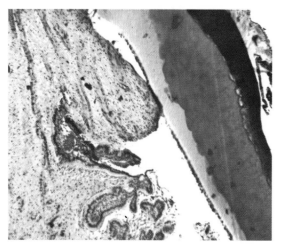

Ameloblastic Fibro-odontoma × 50

(Bottom) The lesion exhibited here is a type of *mixed odontogenic tumor,* with the soft-tissue elements to the left and the hard tissue to the right. The epithelium, proliferating in the connective tissue stroma, shows varying degrees of differentiation in an ameloblastomatous pattern. The purple-staining strip near the right border is enamel matrix that covers the red-staining dentin and lighter predentin. Since there are components of ameloblastic fibroma and odontoma, the term *ameloblastic fibro-odontoma* is applied.

Neoplasms histologically similar to ameloblastoma are found in the pituitary region. They arise from remnants of Rathke's pouch, an invagination of the primitive oral epithelium. Their histogenesis may be explained on the basis that the parent cells had the potential to form an enamel organ. The "ameloblastomas" of the tibia probably are tumors of vascular origin that simulate the pattern of the ameloblastoma.

ODONTOMA

An odontoma, or more specifically a composite (mixed) odontoma, is a tumorous anomaly of calcified dental tissues involving both ectodermal (enamel) and mesodermal (dentin, cementum, pulp) structures. Two types of composite odontomas are recognized: (1) the complex type, which consists of a single mass of dentin, cementum, and enamel in abnormal relation; and (2) the compound type, consisting of several small masses in which the anatomic relation of the dental tissues is such that the structures formed by these tissues are more or less recognizable as rudimentary teeth. Occasionally, features of both types are evident in a single case. In that event the designation of the lesion should be determined by its most predominant characteristic, or it may be referred to as a complex-compound composite odontoma. Because these lesions are limited in growth, they probably are not true neoplasms, as the term *odontoma* would imply.

(Top) Radiograph of part of a large complex composite odontoma in the maxillary molar region. The radiopaque mass surrounded by a radiolucent line is fairly diagnostic of the anomaly. This defect of development may arise from regular or supernumerary tooth buds.

(Center) Illustration of an exposed complex composite odontoma in the mandibular 3rd molar region of a 65-year-old woman, depicting the gross characteristics of this type of odontoma. The emergence of such anomalies is rare. In this patient, its exposure may be attributed to bone resorption in an edentulous area associated with a denture that had been worn for many years.

(Bottom) A photomicrograph from a section of the complex composite odontoma shown at the top of this page. The dental tissues are arranged haphazardly and are not in the form of a tooth. The dense portion composing the bulk of the section is a mixture of dentin and cementum. The various-sized circular areas were filled with enamel, but because of decalcification, only remnants of the enamel matrix are present. The inset shows the enamel pattern from one of these areas at higher magnification. The dental tissues are arranged haphazardly, not in the relationships that are normal in a tooth or developing tooth.

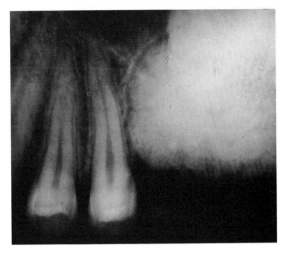

Complex Composite Odontoma

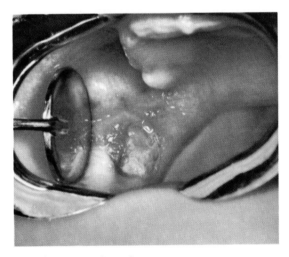

Complex Composite Odontoma

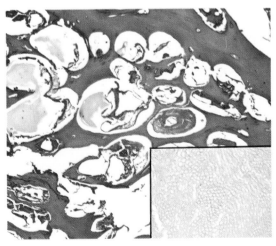

×20   *Complex Composite Odontoma*   ×180

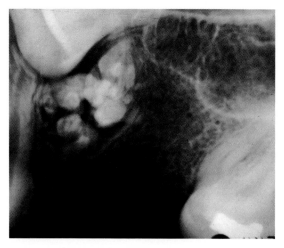

Compound Composite Odontoma

ODONTOMA *(continued)*

(Top) A compound composite odontoma that apparently has prevented the eruption of the permanent premolar. It is composed of numerous small radiopaque masses having the same density as tooth structure. One can be fairly certain of the diagnosis from a radiograph, but histologic examination should be made to rule out neoplastic change. Odontomas usually are removed if they can be expected to interfere with the eruption of normal teeth. They have the same density as normal tooth structure and exhibit the same radiopacity. The compound composite odontoma seen in this radiograph is composed of several small radiopaque masses and apparently has prevented the eruption of the premolar.

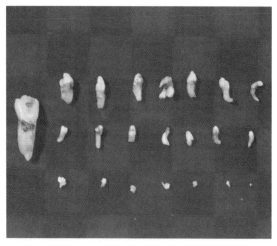

Denticles from Compound Composite Odontoma

(Center) Components of a compound composite odontoma. The structures found in these anomalies may vary in size, number, and configuration. Some of them duplicate specific tooth forms, while others are amorphous masses. As many as 200 such structures have been observed in a single lesion.

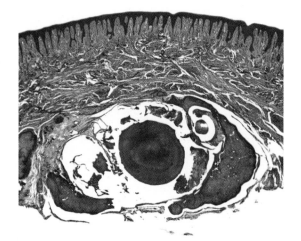

Extraosseous Odontoma ×14

(Bottom) A photomicrograph of a small compound composite anomaly that developed extraosseously. Clinically, this lesion, which was located between the maxillary lateral and central incisors, appeared to be a fibroid hyperplasia. Only upon sectioning was the odontoma discovered. The patient, when a small child, received a severe injury in this region, which may account for the misplaced odontogenic epithelium from which the anomaly developed. Near the upper border of the illustration is surface epithelium of the oral cavity (dark blue). Next is a mass of dense fibrous connective tissue staining a reddish color. In the midst of the connective tissue near the lower border, blue-staining dentin and cementum appear. The partially clear area contains fragments of enamel matrix.

BENIGN FIBRO-OSSEOUS TUMORS

Benign fibro-osseous lesions include several disorders. In all, normal bone is replaced by fibroblasts, collagen fibers, and mineralized tissue. These lesions often arise from cells of the periodontal ligament and have the potential to produce bone, cementum, or a mixture of the two. Radiographically in the early stages these lesions present as circumscribed radiolucencies and become progressively more radiopaque as they mature. Cortical expansion sometimes occurs. Differential diagnosis can be difficult when the lesion is in the radiolucent stage.

(Top) Large, sharply circumscribed lesion involving the body and angle of the mandible. It is radiolucent peripherally and radiopaque centrally. The streaks radiating from the central mass in this case may be suggestive of the "sun-ray" appearance of sarcomas of the jaw bones (see p. 177) but histologic examination revealed that the tumor was composed of fibrous connective tissue and bone, with the latter predominating (ossifying fibroma). Benign fibro-osseous lesions generally grow very slowly in adults. However, when they occur before puberty, they sometimes grow rapidly and produce a marked deformity. Ossifying fibrous tumors in some instances are difficult to distinguish from fibrous dysplasia by microscopic means alone. Radiographic, microscopic, and clinical information are all necessary.

(Center) These lesions may consist of bone, cementum, or fibrous connective tissue in varying proportions. If the predominant product in the lesional tissue is bone, the term *ossifying fibroma* is applied.

(Bottom) Even though one of the products (bone or cementum) may predominate, almost all lesions show a mixture of hard tissue. If there are significant proportions of more than one product, the term *cemento-ossifying fibroma* is applied. The histopathologic terms applied (*ossifying fibroma, cementifying fibroma, cemento-ossifying fibroma*) have little clinical or prognostic significance. Other fibro-osseous lesions are fibrous dysplasia (see p. 126) and familial fibrous dysplasia.

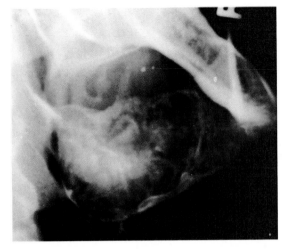

Ossifying Fibroma, Mandible

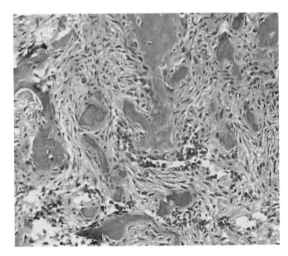

Ossifying Fibroma ×450

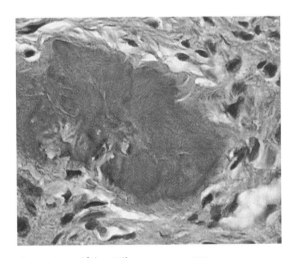

Cemento-ossifying Fibroma ×450

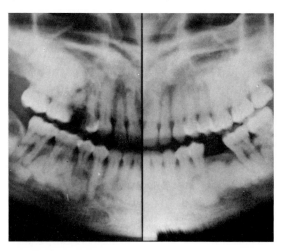

Florid Osseous Dysplasia

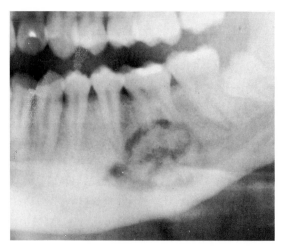

Cementoblastoma, Mandible

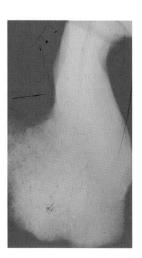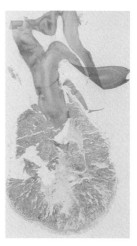

Cementoblastoma, Gross and Microscopic

BENIGN FIBRO-OSSEOUS TUMORS
(continued)

Florid Osseous Dysplasia

(Top) Florid osseous dysplasia is an exuberant multiquadrant process that is microscopically similar to benign fibro-osseous tumors. The World Health Organization (WHO) uses the designation *gigantiform cementoma* for this condition, and also lists the term *familial multiple cementomas* as a synonym. There is constant and marked predisposition for occurrence in black women. The radiographic pattern may change, usually to a more radiopaque character. The disease affects only the alveolar processes and seems independent of teeth. Some cases become complicated by localized osteomyelitis from periodontal disease or periapical inflammation. Traumatic bone cysts (p. 126) have also been reported associated.

Cementoblastoma

(Center) Cementoblastoma is a benign neoplasm of cementoblasts that bears a microscopic resemblance to the osteoblastoma. The characteristic radiographic feature is a well circumscribed, mottled radiopaque mass attached to a tooth root with a radiolucent border. Two thirds of the cases occur in the mandible, with molars being affected about 40% of the time. Most lesions present without pain or swelling.

(Bottom) Microscopically the neoplasm is continuous with root structures with peripheral radiating columns of cementumlike material *(right)*. Active cementoblasts appear at the periphery and between columns. Treatment consists of surgical enucleation. Recurrences have been reported.

BENIGN TUMORS OF SALIVARY GLAND ORIGIN

Pleomorphic Adenoma

Mixed tumors of the major or minor salivary glands are predominantly benign neoplasms containing both epithelial and mesenchymal elements. Only the epithelial portion is neoplastic and the term *pleomorphic adenoma* is preferred to *mixed tumor*. The epithelial component of the tumor may consist of round, polyhedral, elongated, or stellate cells that stain uniformly and are relatively small. These cells may be arranged in strands, islands, ductlike structures, or large masses. The mesenchymal portion of the neoplasm may be composed of fibrous tissue (dense, hyalinized, loosely arranged, or myxomatoid), pseudocartilage, or bone. Either epithelial or connective tissue may predominate, and the tissue pattern may vary greatly in different lesions and in different areas of the same tumor. Pleomorphic adenomas are more frequently encountered in the parotid. The most common oral sites are the lips and palate. Pleomorphic adenomas usually grow very slowly and appear clinically as smooth, spherical enlargements that are asymptomatic and firm to palpation. They tend to recur as the result of incomplete excision or, in some instances, because of multicentric origin.

(Top) Large benign pleomorphic adenoma involving both the hard and the soft palate. It enlarged slowly to its present size in 6 yr. The lesion was quite firm and interfered with swallowing, breathing, and enunciation.

(Center) The spherical enlargement on the left side of the upper lip might be mistaken for a lipoma or mucocele. This lesion, however, was extremely firm, which should make one suspect a tumor. Because of their accessibility to surgery, pleomorphic adenomas of the lip are readily cured. They grow very slowly and usually do not reach a large size.

(Bottom) In this low-power view of a pleomorphic adenoma arising from minor salivary gland tissue in the lip, a portion of the capsule (reddish-staining) may be seen. To the right of this capsule is normal salivary gland tissue and to the left, the tumor.

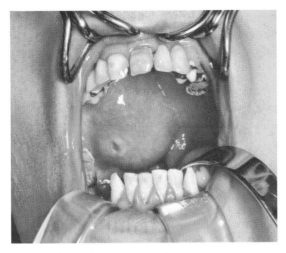

Pleomorphic Adenoma (Mixed Tumor), Palate

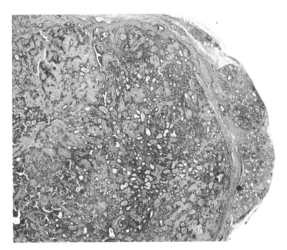

Pleomorphic Adenoma (Mixed Tumor), Lip

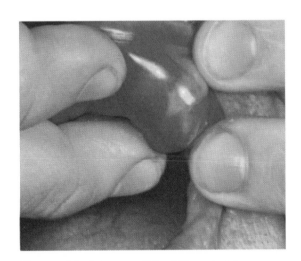

Pleomorphic Adenoma (Mixed Tumor), Lip ×12

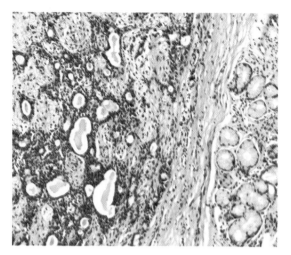

Pleomorphic Adenoma (Mixed Tumor), Lip   × 90

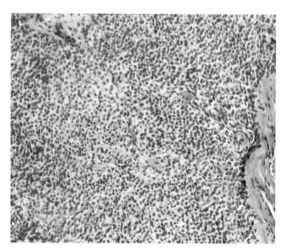

Pleomorphic Adenoma (Mixed Tumor), Cellular Area   × 100

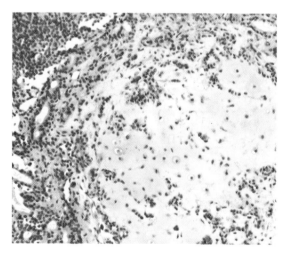

Pleomorphic Adenoma (Mixed Tumor), Pseudocartilaginous Area   × 100

BENIGN TUMORS OF SALIVARY GLAND ORIGIN *(continued)*

(Top) This is a higher magnification of the tumor shown in the last picture on the preceding page. At right is a vertical strip of reddish-staining connective tissue, the tumor capsule. To the right of this capsule several normal mucous acini are apparent. (Compare with those on p. 4.) To the left of the capsule the histologic character of this tumor is demonstrated. It is composed of uniformly dark-staining cuboidal epithelial cells. In some areas these are arranged in a ductal pattern. The epithelial cells in other areas extend from the ducts in strands, and in yet other regions these are clumped in irregular masses. The stroma in this portion of the tumor consists of loosely arranged cellular connective tissue which stains a light blue, due to its myxomatous character.

(Center) It is apparent that this pleomorphic adenoma is quite different histologically from the one in the preceding picture. Here the epithelial component predominates, and the epithelial cells are not in strands, ducts, or islands but are in one large mass. The clinical course of such cellular tumors does not appear to be different from that of the other varieties.

(Bottom) At far left are small, round epithelial cells arranged in islands and ductlike structures. In the remainder of the section is a light-lavender homogeneous substance in which a few cells are entrapped. The tissue in this area resembles hyaline cartilage, especially in regions where an occasional cell has a clear halo about its nucleus. This pseudocartilage is a common finding in pleomorphic adenomas and in some instances may be the predominating feature. Some believe that the hyaline matrix is extravasated epithelial mucin that has widely separated the epithelial cells; others consider it to be a product of myoepithelial cells.

Other benign neoplasms of salivary gland origin include monomorphic adenoma (see p. 163), which is found most often in the upper lip and parotid gland; oxyphilic cell adenoma (oncocytoma), which is characterized by cells with large pink-staining cytoplasm; and Warthin's tumor (see p. 164).

Monomorphic Adenoma

Monomorphic adenomas are benign salivary gland neoplasms in which the neoplastic epithelium is of a regular and uniform type without the diversity that characterizes the histology of pleomorphic adenomas. Further, there is no evidence of the mesenchymal myxochondroid component which is interspersed with the ductal epithelial components of pleomorphic adenomas (see p. 162). Since the histology of individual monomorphic adenomas varies, terms such as *basal cell adenoma, canalicular adenoma, tubular adenoma,* and *trabecular adenoma* are often substituted.

(Top) Monomorphic adenomas may arise in the parotid and other major glands or in the accessory salivary glands in the oral cavity. The upper lip seems to be a favored location for those tumors which arise from accessory salivary glands. Those that are solid will feel firm; some have cystic areas and may feel fluctuant.

(Center) Low-power view of monomorphic adenoma. A capsule is present along the upper margin. There is a single cell type arranged in solid interconnecting nests with minimal supporting stroma.

(Bottom) Monomorphic adenoma showing a canalicular morphology. The long cords of epithelial cells are arranged in a double row. There is a loose fibrillar supporting stroma. Electron microscopic studies have shown that the tall columnar and small basal cells closely resemble those of salivary gland excretory ducts.

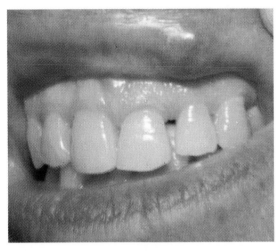

Monomorphic Adenoma, Upper Lip

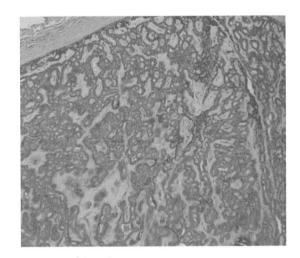

Monomorphic Adenoma × 40

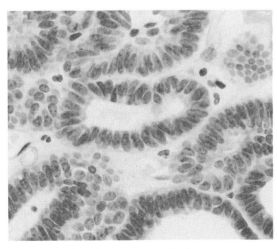

Monomorphic Adenoma, Canalicular Pattern × 100

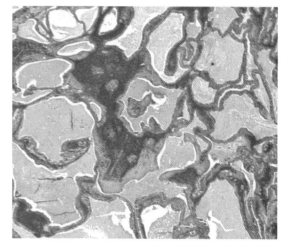

Papillary Cystadenoma Lymphomatosum
(Warthin's Tumor)

BENIGN TUMORS OF SALIVARY GLAND ORIGIN *(continued)*

Papillary Cystadenoma Lymphomatosum

(ADENOLYMPHOMA; WARTHIN'S TUMOR)

(Top) This benign glandular neoplasm (adenoma) occurs in or near the parotid gland. It is probably always benign, although a few questionable exceptions have been reported. Clinically it appears as a slow-growing, hard, nontender lump over the angle or ramus of the mandible or behind the ear. This tumor, which sometimes occurs bilaterally, is much more frequent in males than in females, and its highest incidence is in the 5th decade. The designation *papillary cystadenoma lymphomatosum* is clearly descriptive of the histologic appearance of this entity. The neoplasm has a lymphoid stroma with germinal centers, and the epithelial parenchyma forms tubules and cystic spaces partitioned by numerous papillary projections.

(Center) In this topographic view the lymphoid stroma (dark-blue areas) and numerous large epithelium-lined cysts containing a pink-staining amorphous material are well demonstrated. Papillary projections are seen in a few of the cysts.

Papillary Cystadenoma Lymphomatosum   × 12

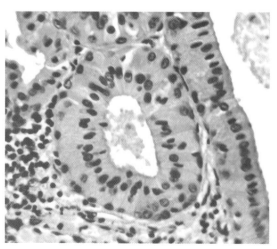

(Bottom) This photomicrograph illustrates the distinctive epithelium of this tumor. The tubule (center) and the microcyst (far right) are lined by large columnar cells with eosinophilic cytoplasm and dark-staining peripherally located nuclei. Toward the basement membrane are one to two rows of cuboid epithelial cells. The most widely accepted theory as to the histogenesis of this neoplasm is that it develops from salivary duct epithelium misplaced in lymph nodes located within or in the vicinity of the parotid. The characteristic epithelial cells in this neoplasm are quite similar to oxyphilic granular cells (oncocytes) found in nonneoplastic salivary gland tissue of individuals over 50 years of age.

Papillary Cystadenoma Lymphomatosum   × 500

MALIGNANT SALIVARY GLAND NEOPLASMS

Malignant neoplasms originating from salivary gland epithelium include the mucoepidermoid carcinoma, the adenoid cystic carcinoma, squamous cell carcinoma, papillary adenocarcinoma, acinic cell adenocarcinoma, acidophilic cell adenocarcinoma, and the so-called malignant mixed tumor (carcinoma in pleomorphic adenoma). Malignant salivary gland neoplasms have high mortality rates. The survival rate depends on the clinical stage (see p. 143), patient age, site, and tumor grade.

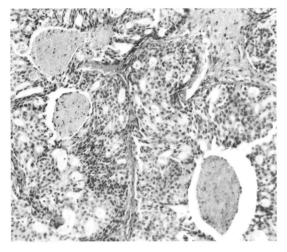

Mucoepidermoid Carcinoma ×100

(Top) The mucoepidermoid carcinoma consists of mucous cells, epidermoid cells, and intermediate cells. These neoplastic cells may be arranged in sheets or islands. They may also form thick-walled, ductlike structures, as seen in this photomicrograph. Mucoepidermoid carcinoma may be subclassified according to degree of malignancy. Those of low-grade malignancy seldom metastasize and have a good prognosis. When considering the diagnosis of mucoepidermoid carcinoma, care must be exercised not to interpret ductal changes due to inflammation (squamous metaplasia and mucous cell proliferation) as being neoplastic.

(Center) A portion of a mucoepidermoid carcinoma showing predominant mucous differentiation. Foci of intermediate cells are situated adjacent to mucus goblet cells near the center.

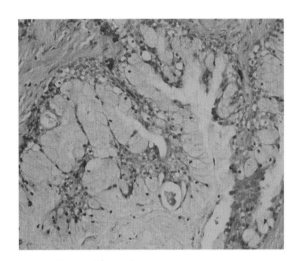

Mucoepidermoid Carcinoma,
Mucous Component ×132

(Bottom) This tumor consists of small, dark-staining cells arranged in groups. In each group are clear areas of various sizes ("Swiss cheese effect"). In other instances there may be anastomosing cords of cells that surround various-sized spaces, dense cords of hyaline stroma separating groups of epithelial cells, or a histologic pattern identical with that of some skin tumors. *Adenoid cystic carcinoma* (pseudoadenomatous basal cell carcinoma, cylindroma, basaloid mixed tumor) is frequently misjudged as being benign. It is a nonencapsulated, slow-growing tumor that is difficult to eradicate. Often there is a history of numerous recurrences with extensive destruction locally. Distant metastases generally occur only late in the disease. Invasion and spread along perineural lymphatics are characteristic of this tumor.

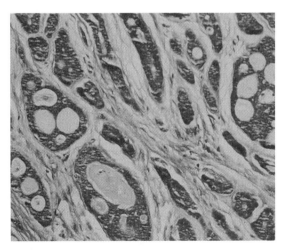

Adenoid Cystic Carcinoma ×132

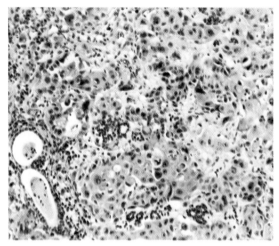

Squamous Cell Carcinoma,
Parotid Gland × 100

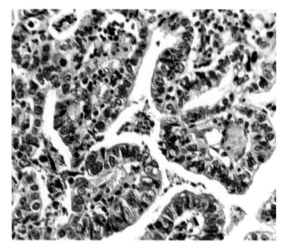

Papillary Adenocarcinoma × 220

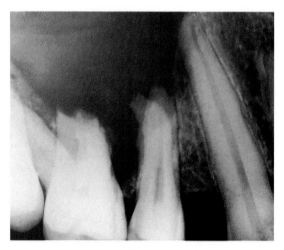

Adenocarcinoma, Maxilla

MALIGNANT SALIVARY GLAND NEOPLASMS *(continued)*

(Top) Except for the two ducts seen near the lower left border, the normal parotid tissue has been replaced completely by malignant squamous cells. These vary in size and shape, and may contain large hyperchromatic nuclei. Squamous cell carcinoma may develop in a pleomorphic adenoma or mucoepidermoid tumor, or directly from metaplastic ductal epithelium.

(Center) This malignant epithelial tumor originated from salivary gland tissue in the floor of the mouth. It is characterized by vascular papillary projections that are bordered by a single row of epithelial cells. These cells vary in size and shape. In some the hyperchromatic nuclei are at one end of the cell, and in others at the opposite end. In certain instances the nuclei are so large that they nearly fill the cells.

The acinic cell adenocarcinoma may be composed of either serous cells (serous cell adenocarcinoma) or mucous cells (mucous or clear cell adenocarcinoma). The acidophilic cell adenocarcinoma (malignant oncocytoma or oxyphilic cell carcinoma) is composed of large cells with reddish-staining cytoplasm somewhat like cells in Warthin's tumor, although not so regularly shaped. The term *malignant mixed tumor* is applied by some practitioners to a cancerous growth of salivary gland tissue that in some areas exhibits qualities of a conventional mixed tumor, or where a malignancy develops in a long-standing pleomorphic adenoma. Others prefer to designate such a lesion according to its malignant component (*e.g.*, adenocarcinoma or squamous cell carcinoma) and limit the use of "mixed tumor" to benign lesions.

(Bottom) Radiographic appearance of a maxilla that was invaded by an adenocarcinoma of salivary gland origin. It is apparent that, in addition to the extensive bone destruction, the mesial and lingual roots of the 1st molar have been irregularly resorbed, leaving spikelike projections. Whenever "spiking" of the roots is seen, the diagnostician should suspect a malignant lesion.

BASAL CELL CARCINOMA

Basal cell carcinoma usually arises from the basal cells of the epidermis, but it may originate from the outermost cells of hair follicles or sebaceous glands. It may occur anywhere in skin but is most common on the upper part of the face. It grows very slowly and rarely metastasizes. It may be cured readily by excision or radiation therapy. If left untreated, it may destroy the face and invade the underlying bone and cartilage. This neoplasm may extend into the oral or ocular mucous membranes but rarely originates in these areas. This lesion is the least malignant of all cancerous growths, and—except in very advanced cases—the prognosis is excellent. It is most common in males with light-colored skin that has become dry and atrophic from exposure to wind and sunlight.

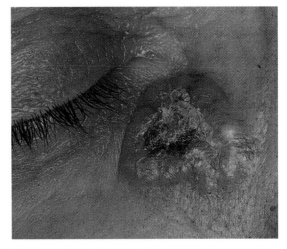

Basal Cell Carcinoma, Cheek

(Top) This basal cell carcinoma is a raised, waxy, slightly ulcerated lesion that reached its present size in 3 years. It usually begins as a small papule with a scaly surface. The patient may believe it is a "pimple" that is slow to heal because the scab comes off continually. Basal cell carcinoma at this stage may be differentiated clinically from an inflammatory lesion by its very thin, threadlike, raised, pearly border with central necrosis.

(Center) Typical microscopic appearance of basal cell carcinoma. The malignant epithelial cells are oval or cylindrical and have deeply staining nuclei. These cells are arranged in islands of various sizes and shapes. At the periphery of each island there is a single row of radically oriented cells. This regimented arrangement is best seen at upper left. At upper right the origin is evident.

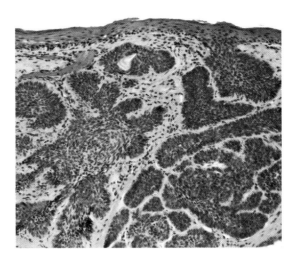

Basal Cell Carcinoma × 100

NEVOID BASAL CELL CARCINOMA SYNDROME

(Bottom) This 13-year-old boy had basal cell lesions about both eyes. Microscopically, they were similar to the lesion in the center picture. Keratin-filled cysts in the jaws were enucleated on several occasions. Removal of carcinomas and cysts as they occur is a continuing but essential treatment. The syndrome consists of multiple basal cell carcinomas, keratocysts of the jaws, bifid ribs, vertebral anomalies, pitted palms, and other defects.

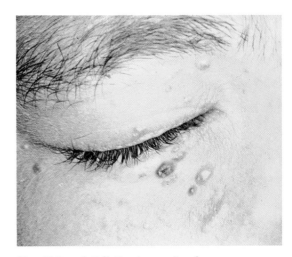

Nevoid Basal Cell Carcinoma Syndrome

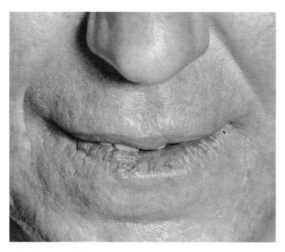

Carcinoma, Lip

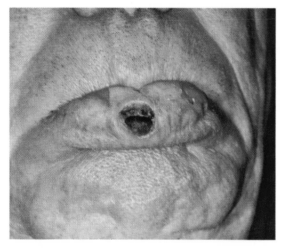

Carcinoma, Lip

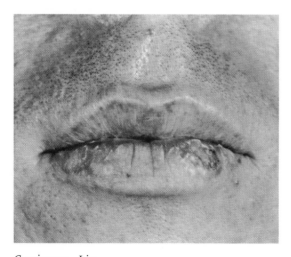

Carcinoma, Lip

SQUAMOUS CELL CARCINOMA

Squamous cell carcinomas of the oral cavity usually are moderately well differentiated neoplasms. In general, they are more frequent in men than in women. The prognosis varies according to the location, but the 5-year survival rate for each area depends on how early in the disease proper treatment is instituted. Oral carcinoma may appear as a keratotic plaque; a crusted ulcer; a noncrusted ulcer, either superficial or deep; a slightly raised lesion with central ulceration and a rolled border; a slightly raised red lesion; a red velvety area; or a verruciform growth.

(Top) Stage I carcinoma in the lower lip, on the vermilion border about halfway between the commissure and the midline. It may begin as a keratotic plaque, as shown here, or as a crusted ulcer that might be mistaken for herpes labialis. Metastasis, which occurs first to the submental lymph nodes, is not an early finding. The prognosis is very good unless the lesion is extensive.

(Center) Stage II carcinoma. The carcinoma in this instance is a sharply circumscribed, crusted ulcer. On each side of the lesion atrophic changes similar to those seen in solar cheilosis are evident. The surgical treatment of such a case should include vermilionectomy as a prophylactic measure.

(Bottom) Stage II carcinoma. This lesion is slightly elevated above the surface, and it has a characteristic firm, rolled border. Unless a carcinoma is in an extremely early stage, it is not possible to get the fingers under it when attempting to lift it up. Carcinoma of the lower lip is principally a disease of men. It is rare in blacks. It usually occurs during the 6th decade but is not uncommon in much younger individuals. Solar cheilosis is often a predisposing change, as here.

Carcinoma in the upper lip has a low incidence. It may metastasize to the upper cervical, preauricular, or submandibular lymph nodes. It grows more rapidly than carcinoma of the lower lip, and its prognosis is not so good.

The second most frequent site of oral carcinoma is the tongue (the most frequent intraoral site is the floor of the mouth). Squamous cell carcinoma involving the tongue usually arises in the middle third of the lateral border or on the ventral surface. It is relatively rare on the tip and dorsum. Carcinomas of the tongue metastasize very early, usually to the submandibular group of lymph nodes. Proper treatment must be instituted while the lesion is still small if a long survival period is to be anticipated. Procrastination in biopsying and treating a suspicious lesion may result in a needless fatality.

(Top) Stage IV carcinoma. Typical appearance of a moderately advanced squamous cell carcinoma on the lateral border of the tongue. The periphery of the lesion is raised, rolled, and firm. The central portion is ulcerated and has a granular appearance.

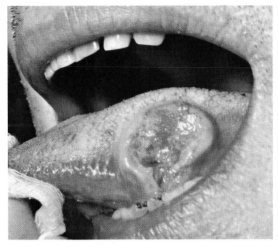

Carcinoma, Tongue

(Center) Stage III carcinoma. This ulcerated lesion in the floor of the mouth proved on biopsy to be squamous cell carcinoma. Note the adjacent erythroplakia which extends medially from the ulcer. Because cancer in its early stages is not painful, many lesions that are not readily visible to the patient are not detected until they are fairly extensive. Therefore the best opportunity to detect intraoral cancer early is afforded to practitioners making routine oral examinations.

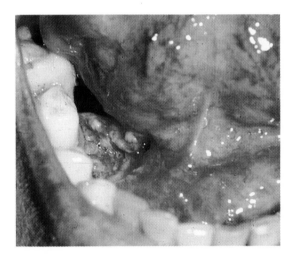

Carcinoma, Floor of Mouth

(Bottom) Stage IV carcinoma. The floor of the mouth is currently the most common site for development of intraoral carcinoma. Most lesions appear as ulcerations, some extending to the ventral surface of the tongue. Nonulcerated lesions may appear as firm swellings with a red granular surface. Biopsy is essential for diagnosis.

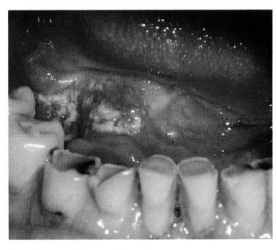

Carcinoma, Floor of Mouth

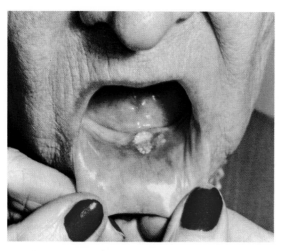

Carcinoma, Alveolar Mucosa

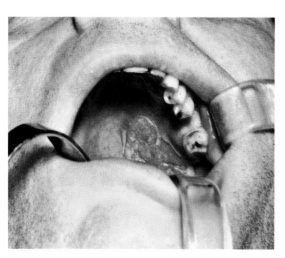

Carcinoma, Palate

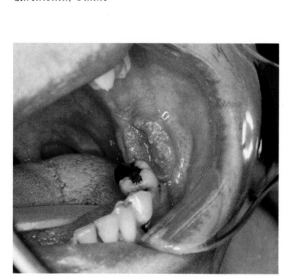

Carcinoma, Retromolar Region

SQUAMOUS CELL CARCINOMA
(continued)

(Top) Stage I carcinoma. This carcinomatous lesion involving the alveolar ridge and the vestibular mucosa is bisected by a groove. This groove was produced by pressure from a denture flange. Inflammatory lesions that are fissured and ulcerated are frequently observed in patients wearing ill-fitting dentures. Such lesions may appear somewhat similar to the carcinoma shown here. If they do not disappear quickly after the denture is trimmed, they should be biopsied.

(Center) Stage III carcinoma. This squamous cell carcinoma of the palate appears as an ulcer with slightly raised, rolled edges. Palatal carcinoma is relatively common in countries where cigars and cigarettes frequently are smoked by putting the lighted end in the mouth. Carcinoma of the floor of the mouth (which must be suspected early and treated adequately) often appears as a shallow but extensive ulcer not unlike this palatal lesion. Some carcinomas of the palate and buccal mucosa are papillomatous and well differentiated. These lesions are more common in males. There is metastasis to cervical nodes in about one-fifth of the patients. The 5-year survival for Stage I lesions is about 70%, declining to about 6% for Stage IV lesions.

(Bottom) Stage III carcinoma. A large carcinoma in the retromolar region and buccal mucosa appears as an ulcer with a heavy distinct rolled border. The patient did not notice it until it was large enough to impinge on the upper jaw when occluding.

Oral carcinoma may simulate other disease processes and vice versa. Therefore, if too much reliance is placed on the clinical characteristics, many incipient carcinomatous lesions will be overlooked. Some mucous membrane carcinomas are not ulcerated but appear as red, raised, innocent-looking lesions. It is good practice to take a biopsy of every lesion of over 2-wk duration, the exact nature of which is not known. There is no harm in biopsying a lesion that proves to be noncancerous. Any disadvantage associated with biopsy of a cancerous lesion is far outweighed by the advantage of establishing the diagnosis. The time between microscopic diagnosis and definitive treatment should be minimal.

(Top) Carcinoma *in situ* (intraepithelial carcinoma) may appear at the edge of an infiltrating carcinoma or may be the only mucosal change in the area. It is characterized by malignant changes that are limited to the epithelium. It may eventually become invasive. The photomicrograph includes the junction between normal epithelium (far right) and carcinoma *in situ*. To the right of center there is an abrupt change in the character of the epithelium. To the left of this area the cells are not in normal relationship. There is an increased number of cells as well as alteration in their character. The nuclei are variable in size and hyperchromatic. The basal layer, however, is intact. The epithelial changes in carcinoma *in situ* are somewhat similar to those in epithelial dysplasia, except that they are more extensive.

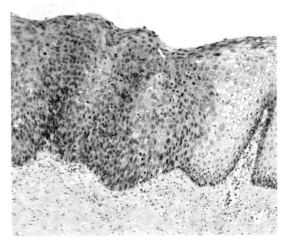

Carcinoma in Situ × 100

(Center) Relatively well differentiated squamous cell carcinoma is demonstrated in this photomicrograph. In the upper left corner there is a segment of surface epithelium that is relatively normal. The squamous epithelium in the rest of the photomicrograph is carcinomatous. It shows loss of organization. The cells are large, with abundant light-blue-staining cytoplasm. Properly oriented basal cells are not evident at the periphery. At lower left is a strand of epithelium containing circumscribed nests of cells that have abundant eosinophilic cytoplasm and pyknotic nuclei.

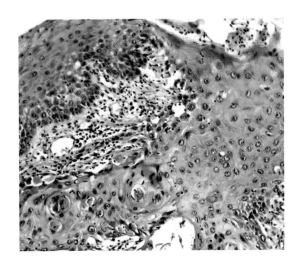

Squamous Cell Carcinoma × 150

(Bottom) At top center the covering epithelium is thin, nonpapillated, and hyperkeratotic. The subepithelial connective tissue is infiltrated heavily with inflammatory cells. In the center of the photomicrograph is a large, circular, laminated hyaline structure surrounded by epithelial cells. This is a so-called epithelial pearl. Such structures are commonly found in moderately well differentiated squamous cell carcinoma. To the right of this central mass and at the far left are nests of atypical epithelial cells. Below the pearl are other malignant cells that are somewhat difficult to recognize because of the heavy inflammatory infiltrate.

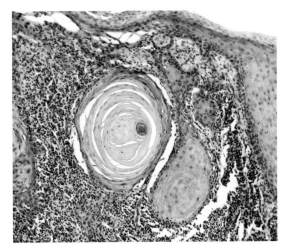

Squamous Cell Carcinoma, Epithelial Pearl
× 80

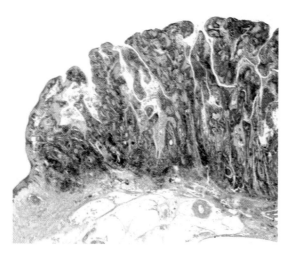

Squamous Cell Carcinoma, Verrucous Type　×7

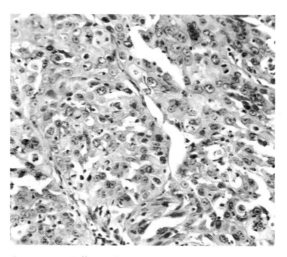

Squamous Cell Carcinoma　×180

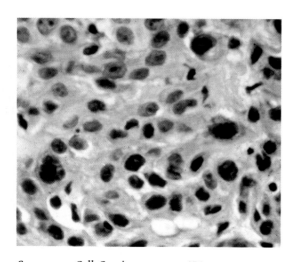

Squamous Cell Carcinoma　×450

SQUAMOUS CELL CARCINOMA
(continued)

(Top) Low-power view of a verrucous or papillomatous squamous cell carcinoma of 1 year's duration. At far left is normal surface epithelium. The numerous projecting structures are composed of atypical epithelial cells (not apparent at this magnification). Keratohyalin and cellular debris are entrapped between the fingerlike projections. It is apparent that this carcinoma has not invaded deeply; much of it extends above the normal mucosal level. Clinically it might have been confused with a papilloma, wart, or keratoacanthoma. Carcinomas growing in a verrucal pattern tend to be fairly well differentiated lesions. In some instances the diagnosis may be missed microscopically if the pathologist is not given sufficient material to examine. Verruciform carcinomas generally have a better prognosis than other types, but this advantage may be offset somewhat by the fact that their true nature is not always suspected clinically until they have reached a large size.

(Center) Some of the characteristic alterations observed in squamous cell carcinoma are demonstrated in this photomicrograph. Nearly all of the cells are large, with abundant, light-staining cytoplasm. There is much variation in nuclear form and in staining characteristics. Many nuclei are vesicular and have distinct nucleoli. In some cells the chromatin material is compact and stains intensely. There are numerous mitotic figures, some of which are abnormal. Several atypical mitotic figures can be seen near the upper right corner. To the left and above these are a few cells with vesicular nuclei and prominent nucleoli. Large, bizarre cells are apparent at the lower right and left.

(Bottom) A portion of a poorly differentiated (anaplastic) squamous cell carcinoma. It is apparent that there is a marked variation in nuclear size and pattern. Near the right border are several large, bizarre nuclear masses. A similar mass is seen at lower left. Three pyknotic chromatin masses are seen near the upper right corner. The nuclei in some of the cells are pale-staining but have prominent nucleoli. The cell boundaries in many instances are indistinct.

(Top) The nodular enlargement of the lateral neck, outlined with indelible pencil, is a lymph node invaded by carcinoma metastatic from the oral cavity. Squamous cell carcinoma almost always metastasizes by the lymphatic route. Knowledge of the lymph drainage of the tumor site will enable one to anticipate which lymph nodes may become involved. Enlargement of lymph nodes in adults, unless obviously related to inflammatory disease, or to lymphoma (see p. 175), should be considered the result of metastatic cancer until proven otherwise.

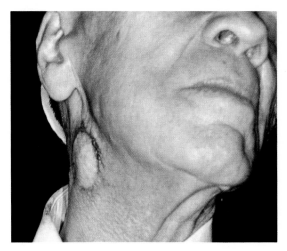

Metastatic Carcinoma, Cervical Lymph Node

(Center) Squamous cell carcinoma that has metastasized to a lymph node. Some of the lymph node architecture is still discernible. At far left is a circular mass of lymphocytes that is a germinal center (lymphoid follicle). In the rest of the photomicrograph are neoplastic epithelial cells that are characterized by moderately abundant cytoplasm and large pleomorphic nuclei. Lymphocytes are scattered among the malignant cells. In some instances an entire node will be replaced by neoplastic tissue.

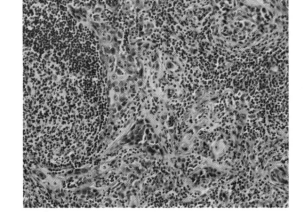

Metastatic Squamous Cell Carcinoma $\times 100$

CARCINOMA OF THE NASOPHARYNX

(Bottom) Carcinomas arising in the nasopharynx have a tendency to remain small and symptomless at their primary site. Frequently the first obvious manifestation of the disease is metastatic lymphadenopathy, as shown here. This patient, who was referred for dental examination, had no complaints except for the asymptomatic swelling near the angle of the mandible. This had been present for 3 mo and had not responded to antibiotic therapy. Clinical and radiographic examination did not reveal any disease process in the oral cavity that might be related to the enlarged lymph nodes. The oral diagnostician, being cognizant of the peculiarities of cancer of the nasopharynx, suggested that this region be examined for neoplastic disease. A very small lesion was discovered which proved to be a nonkeratinizing squamous cell carcinoma (see p. 174). Despite intensive radiation therapy, the disease proved fatal in 12 mo, with widespread metastases.

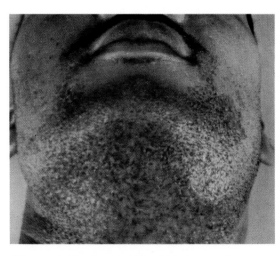

Metastatic Nonkeratinizing Squamous Cell Carcinoma, Left Cervical Nodes

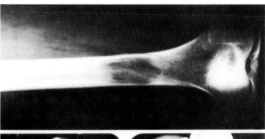

*Nonkeratinizing Squamous Cell
Carcinoma* × 500

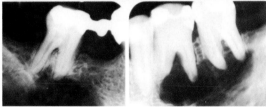

Multiple Myeloma, Femur and Mandible

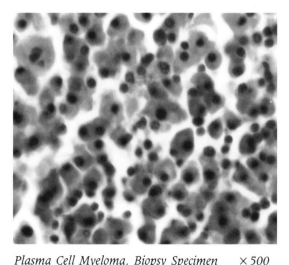

Plasma Cell Myeloma, Biopsy Specimen × 500

CARCINOMA OF THE NASOPHARYNX
(continued)

(Top) Histologic appearance of a nonkeratinizing carcinoma (formerly termed *lymphoepithelioma* or *Schmincke tumor*). Near the center and the lower border are several large oval or circular structures. These are nuclei of malignant epithelial cells. Each contains at least one large nucleolus. Such nucleoli have some affinity for eosin and may stain slightly red. The borders of the epithelial cells are very indistinct. Scattered among these cells, and also in the adjacent tissue, are several lymphocytes. These lesions have also been termed *transitional cell carcinomas.* When in the palate these neoplasms have a tendency to spread locally.

PLASMA-CELL MYELOMA

(MULTIPLE MYELOMA)

Plasma-cell myeloma, a malignant tumor that primarily involves the bone marrow, is characterized by a slow but progressive destruction of skeletal parts. Its highest incidence is after the 4th decade, and it occurs in men more frequently than in women. The bone lesions, which are sharply outlined, contain closely packed cells that resemble plasma cells. Most, but not all, cases are characterized by Bence Jones protein in the urine. Serum electrophoresis will reveal abnormal M-type protein, usually IgG.

(Center) The radiolucent areas in the molar regions were discovered when radiographs were taken to determine the cause of pain in the mandible. A skeletal survey revealed "punched-out" lesions in many of the bones, one of which appears at the top of this illustration. Occasionally, a spontaneous fracture of an involved weight-bearing bone may be the first indication of this disease. Within the jaws the lesions in their early stages may resemble periapical pathoses.

(Bottom) Moderately compact mass of cells, many of which closely resemble plasma cells (see p. 8). Care must be exercised not to make the diagnosis of myeloma based on the presence of a mass of plasma cells in granulation tissue. In multiple myeloma there is some degree of pleomorphism, the cells are closely packed, and stroma is very scant.

MALIGNANT LYMPHOMA

Malignant lymphoma is an inclusive term for neo-plasms arising from lymphoid tissue. Malignant lymphomas consist of Hodgkin's disease and the non-Hodgkin's lymphomas. In the latter category are neoplasms of the lymphocytic series (lympho-cytic lymphomas), such as small cell, large cell, lymphoblastic, and follicular types and mixed lym-phomas. Tumors formerly identified as *histiocytic lymphomas* are generally regarded to be of lympho-cytic origin. Burkitt's lymphoma occurs endemically in the jaws of African children but is observed spo-radically in other regions of the world. It may be caused by Epstein-Barr virus (EBV). Malignant lymphomas arise most often in major lymph nodes such as those in the neck, axilla, mediastinum, and groin. They also can arise from extranodal lymphoid tissue and can arise within bone.

(Top) Enlargement of lymph nodes in lymphocy-tic lymphoma. The large nodular mass in the supra-clavicular region was nontender and moderately firm to palpation. A small lump was noted in this area 6 wk previously. The patient died 9 wk after the first clinical manifestations of the disease.

(Center) Large cell lymphoma cells predominate in this section. They have large nuclei in which the chromatin particles are widely dispersed. The nuclei are also somewhat vesicular rather than solid. The prognosis of a given lymphoma relates to the his-tologic type, immunologic typing, and degree of systemic involvement at the time of diagnosis.

(Bottom) Hodgkin's disease is characterized histo-logically by the presence of Dorothy Reed (Reed-Sternberg) cells. In the photomicrograph several of these special cells are seen. At the left is one with a trilobed nucleus (due to fusion of three cells); others are apparent at the right.

Clinical staging is important in managing patients with Hodgkin's disease. In Stage I, where the disease is limited to one anatomic area and has not crossed the diaphragm, it is, for all practical purposes, cur-able using radiation therapy, chemotherapy, or a combination of the two.

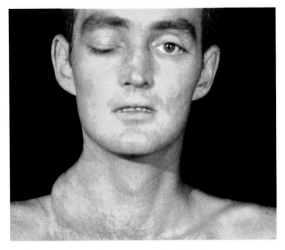

Malignant Lymphoma, Cervical Nodes

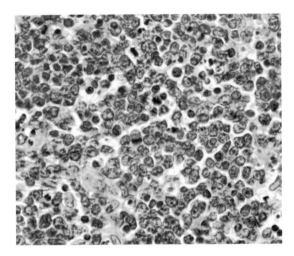

Large Cell Lymphoma   ×400

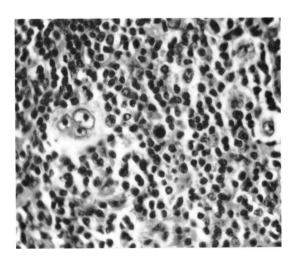

Hodgkin's Disease, Reed-Sternberg Cells   ×350

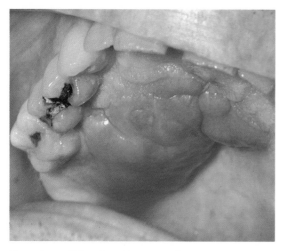

Lymphoproliferative Disease, Palate

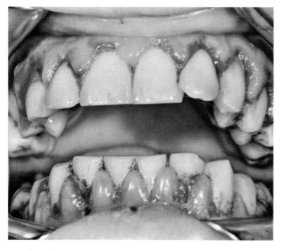

Leukemia

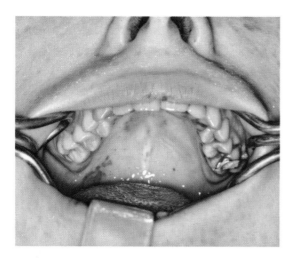

Leukemia

MALIGNANT LYMPHOMA *(continued)*

(Top) *Lymphoproliferative disease* is a term applied to malignant lymphomas that arise in extranodal lymphoid tissues, such as in the palatal salivary glands or Waldeyer's ring. At the time of diagnosis there is usually no involvement of any major lymph nodes, the disease being confined to the local area. In the case illustrated, the disease was confined to the palatal tissue. Differential diagnosis would include dental infection, salivary gland neoplasm, or a neoplasm extending from the maxillary sinus. Definitive diagnosis requires biopsy.

LEUKEMIA

Leukemias are a group of disorders with the common feature of unregulated proliferation in the bone marrow of a member of the white blood cell series. Leukemic cells overgrow and replace normal marrow elements and appear in the peripheral blood. Leukemia may be designated lymphocytic, monocytic, and granulocytic (myelocytic), indicating the histogenesis of the neoplasm. Each case of leukemia may be designated as acute or chronic. The acute is characterized by poorly differentiated cells, and the chronic type by well-differentiated cells. In general, the more differentiated the cells, the longer the course of the disease. The oral changes that may occur in leukemia are related to local leukemic infiltrations, thrombocytopenia, neutropenia, and anemia.

(Center) The gingival tissue in this leukemic patient is enlarged in many areas due to an infiltration of the abnormal cells (see leukemic gingivitis, p. 77). Another common oral manifestation of leukemia, gingival hemorrhage, is also apparent. This patient was not aware of the leukemia when appearing for dental care until a blood count was done.

(Bottom) In this leukemic patient the mucosa is pale, and numerous petechiae are seen in the hard and soft palates as well as in the lip. In some cases minor acts of trauma may produce ulcers that will not heal due to the diminished number of circulating neutrophils (see agranulocytosis, p. 139).

OSTEOGENIC SARCOMA

In osteogenic sarcoma, which is a malignant neoplasm of bone-forming mesenchymal tissue, the bone usually is produced directly from the tumor parenchyma, but some may be formed from cartilage. This neoplasm is highly malignant and generally metastasizes to the lungs by the vascular route. Osteogenic sarcomas occur most frequently in the 2nd and 3rd decades. They occur about equally in the maxilla and mandible. They are relatively rare in older individuals except in patients with Paget's disease (see p. 129).

(Top) Osteogenic sarcoma in the left mandible of a 19-year-old male. Biting on this large nodular mass caused it to become distorted and ulcerated.

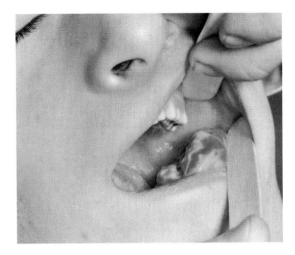

Osteogenic Sarcoma, Mandible

(Center) Two areas from a single tumor are demonstrated in this photomicrograph. At left is proliferating connective tissue in which there are atypical spindle and stellate cells. At right, near the lower border, atypical bone is being formed directly from the malignant connective tissue.

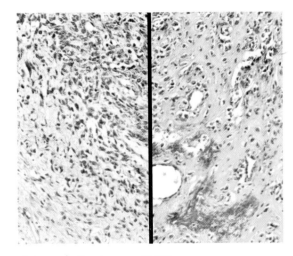

Osteogenic Sarcoma × 100

CHONDROSARCOMA

Chondrosarcoma is a malignant neoplasm of mesenchymal tissue that produces atypical, poorly differentiated cartilage. Some bone may be produced in the neoplasm and develops directly from the connective tissue along with the cartilage. Chondrosarcoma is most prevalent in individuals 30 to 50 years of age, does not generally run a rapid course except in the jaws, and in many instances appears to develop from preexisting benign cartilaginous tumors.

(Bottom) This chondrosarcoma in the maxilla is radiopaque centrally and radiolucent peripherally. The "sun-ray" appearance resulting from the radiopaque streaks extending from the central calcified mass commonly is considered characteristic of sclerosing osteogenic sarcoma. Histologic examination revealed a cartilaginous tumor with a marked amount of calcification and ossification. It appeared benign and was diagnosed as an osteochondroma. There was massive recurrence 4 years later, at which time biopsy revealed chondrosarcoma. Upon further sectioning and reevaluation of the first biopsy specimen, small sarcomatous areas were discovered.

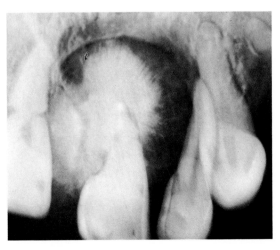

Chondrosarcoma

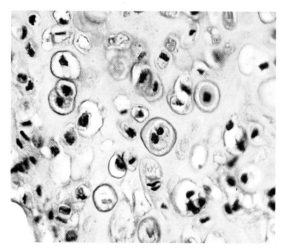

Chondrosarcoma ×220

CHONDROSARCOMA *(continued)*

(Top) In some chondrosarcomas histologic evidence of malignancy is readily apparent. In many, however, most of the cartilage cells are well differentiated, and malignant characteristics may be overlooked unless sufficient material is examined in detail. A cartilaginous neoplasm should be considered malignant if in some areas the following are apparent: large nuclei, some binucleated cells, and occasional large cells with several nuclei or clumped chromatin. In the accompanying photomicrograph all these malignant features are apparent.

Some pathologists designate malignant bone- or cartilage-producing tumors according to the main component or components. Others classify all such neoplasms as osteosarcomas.

FIBROSARCOMA

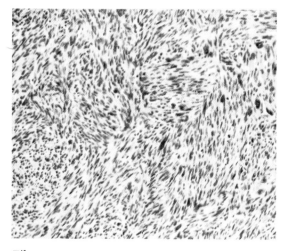

Fibrosarcoma ×100

(Center) Fibrosarcoma is a malignant neoplasm of fibroblasts. It may arise from the periosteum or from extraosseous soft tissue. The aggressiveness of these tumors varies, but generally they are relatively slow-growing. Many fibrosarcomas are well-differentiated lesions. The one in the photomicrograph, however, is highly anaplastic. It is composed of spindle-shaped cells with hyperchromatic nuclei, many of which are exceptionally large. Throughout the specimen there are bands of tissue in which the cells are oriented in one direction, giving them a combed appearance. Some of these bands are at right angles to others. Malignant tumors of nerve or muscle may sometimes appear quite similar to this lesion. When the tissue of origin is not evident in neoplasms having such a histologic pattern, it is convenient to designate them as *spindle cell sarcomas*.

(Bottom) This is a higher magnification of the tumor in the center picture, showing the component cells in greater detail. It is apparent that most of the cells are spindle-shaped but of various sizes. In several, the chromatin material is irregularly dispersed throughout the nucleus; in other cells it is condensed and stains intensely. At upper right two very large, bizarre chromatin masses are seen.

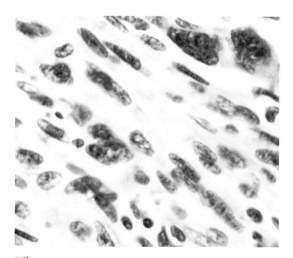

Fibrosarcoma ×575

MELANOMA

(Top)　A melanoma (melanoblastoma, melanocarcinoma) is a neoplasm composed of malignant melanocytes (melanoblasts). It has the potential to metastasize early and widely. Melanoma in the skin and mucous membrane usually appears clinically as an enlarging bluish-black or slate-gray, raised lesion. The pigmented areas seen in the accompanying picture are metastatic lesions. Melanoma is seldom primary in the oral cavity.

Melanomas should be differentiated from pigmented nevi, which are benign. The latter lesions are relatively static, may be raised or flat, and are generally brown except for those designated as blue nevi. The histologic characteristics of the different types are as follows: junctional nevus—clumps of loosened, pigmented cells in the basal cell layer; intradermal nevus—nevus cells grouped in the lamina propria; compound nevus—combination of junctional and intradermal types; blue nevus—heavily pigmented spindle cells deep in the connective tissue. In many instances melanomas appear to have developed from junctional or compound nevi. The first clinical indication of malignant change is an increase in size and in the degree of pigmentation.

(Center)　In the intradermal nevus at left the nevus cells form a solid sheet in the lamina propria, though they are usually found in nests and cords. They are separated from the flattened covering epithelium by a small band of connective tissue. The superficial cells are heavily pigmented. At right is a section from a malignant lesion. The so-called junctional change (loosening of the cells), is evident in the overlying epithelium. In the lamina propria are large, lightly pigmented cells with bizarre nuclei. These are malignant melanocytes that appear to have arisen from within the basal cell layer of the epithelium. The junctional change is not present in metastatic lesions.

(Bottom)　In this melanoma the malignant cells are heavily pigmented. When melanin is not present (amelanotic melanoma), the diagnosis is somewhat difficult. If one suspects melanoma but the biopsy is negative the biopsy should be repeated as long as suspicion persists. Juvenile melanomas, which occur before puberty, appear malignant histologically but do not metastasize.

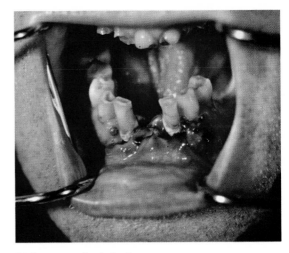

Melanoma, Oral Cavity

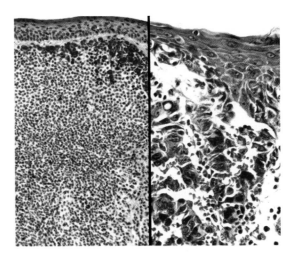

Nevus, Buccal　　　*Melanoma*　×200
Mucosa　×100

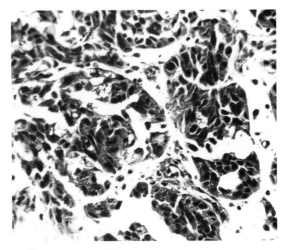

Melanoma　×250

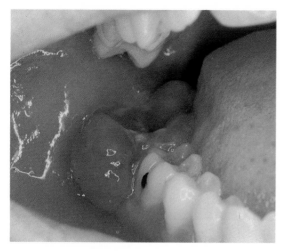

Metastatic Osteosarcoma

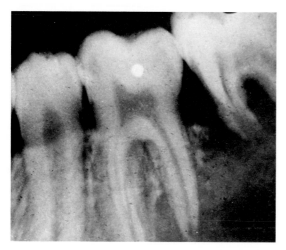

Metastatic Osteosarcoma

METASTASIS TO THE JAWS

Epithelial neoplasms, especially adenocarcinoma, have a marked tendency to metastasize to bone. This is particularly true of adenocarcinomas of breast, thyroid, and prostate, and of hypernephroma. The jaws, especially the mandible, may be the site of intraosseous metastasis. This should always be considered in the patient with a history of previous treatment of malignant neoplasm. Skeletal metastasis may be late, and the lesions may therefore, occur more than 5 years after treatment, when it appears that the primary neoplasm has been treated successfully.

(Top) Metastatic osteosarcoma in a 16-year-old boy appearing as a swelling in the mandibular molar region. Seven months earlier a diagnosis of osteogenic sarcoma was made and the leg amputated. The painless nontender mass was of rubbery consistency and attached to the gingival mucosa distal to and over the 2nd molar.

(Center) Radiographic examination of this patient showed loss of the architecture of the bone surrounding the mandibular 2nd molar and loss of lamina dura distal to the 1st molar. The 2nd molar, which was loose, showed "spiking" of the roots. Looseness of permanent teeth and spiking of the roots should lead to suspicion of malignancy. Infiltration of the right shoulder was also observed radiographically. The 2nd molar showed metastatic tumor in the pulp.

(Bottom) Radiograph showing destruction of alveolar crest by metastatic neoplasm. The irregular pattern of destruction is typical of metastatic neoplasm. Teeth, when present in the area, usually show root resorption with a "spiked" appearance.

Neoplasms may metastasize to the jaws from the thyroid, kidney, breast, bone, lung, colon, prostate, and other sites. The metastatic lesions may appear as diffuse destruction by osteolytic action, as illustrated here, or as cystlike lesions, as illustrated on the following page.

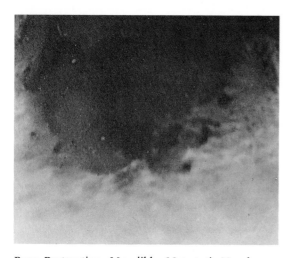

Bone Destruction, Mandible, Metastatic Neoplasm

(Top) This patient had pain, numbness, and looseness of the mandibular teeth. The lateral jaw film shows radiolucencies suggesting the pattern seen in osteomyelitis, multiple myeloma, eosinophilic granuloma, metastatic carcinoma, and possibly ameloblastoma. The patient had been treated for a carcinoma of the prostate, and biopsy of the jaw verified that this was a carcinoma metastatic from the prostate. The history is useful in giving a clue to the primary site; however, the pattern of the primary tumor is reflected in the metastasis and the histologic picture usually is definitive.

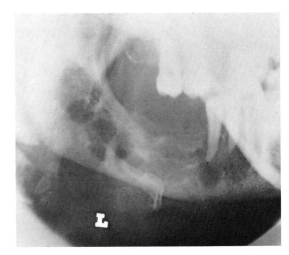

Metastatic Prostatic Carcinoma

(Center) Patient complained of swelling in the region of the angle of the mandible. Lateral jaw films demonstrated a unilocular cystic-appearing lesion at the angle of the mandible. This was misinterpreted as an odontogenic cyst. At surgery it was found to be a solid lesion. Histologic examination demonstrated the lesion was a malignant lymphoma. Other bones had no evidence of tumor. (see p. 175). Lymphomas primary in bone were formerly termed *reticulum cell sarcoma.*

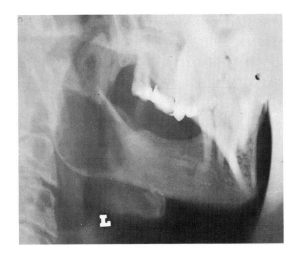

Bone Destruction, Mandible, Malignant Lymphoma

(Bottom) A 9-year-old child had had a diagnosis of neuroblastoma of the adrenal. Metastasis to the bones was widespread, and the jaws did not escape. The 1st molar shown was very loose, and radiographs revealed a "spiking" of the incompletely formed roots, and complete loss of the lamina dura and of the normal architecture of the supporting bone. The loss of bone extends to the 2nd deciduous molar. Whenever a loose permanent tooth is encountered in a young child without evident history of trauma, a malignant neoplasm, either local or metastatic, should be suspected.

Malignant neoplasms are characterized by their ability to metastasize through either the blood or the lymph stream. While classically carcinomas metastasize through lymph channels and sarcomas through blood vessels, there is no hard-and-fast rule. Rarely, tumors may metastasize by transplantation; for example, when cells from an ovarian tumor become detached and spread through the peritoneal cavity, or those from an intraoral tumor are aspirated and become implanted in the lung. Metastasis can occur from the jaws or to the jaws.

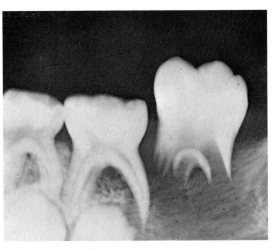

Metastatic Neuroblastoma

Anomalies of Teeth and Selected Genetic Conditions

British Dental Association: The Report on Odontomes. London, John Bale, Sons and Danielsson, Ltd. 1914

Escobar V, Goldblatt L, Bixler, D: A clinical, genetic, and ultrastructural study of snowcapped teeth: Amelogenesis imperfecta, hypomaturation type. Oral Surg Oral Med Oral Pathol 52:607, 1981

Gardner DG, Sapp JP: Regional odontodysplasia. Oral Surg 31:351, 1973

Grover P, Lorton L: Gemination and twinning in the permanent dentition. Oral Surg Oral Med Oral Pathol 59:313, 1985

Mjösir IA: The structure of taurodont teeth. J Dent Child 42:459, 1972

Ruprecht A, Batniji S, El-Neweihi E: The incidence of taurodontism in dental patients. Oral Surg Oral Med Oral Pathol 63:743, 1987

Sclare R: Hereditary opalescent dentin (dentinogenesis imperfecta). Br Dent J 84:164, 1984

Stewart RE, Dixon GH, Graber RB: Dens evaginatus (tuberculated cusps): Genetic and treatment considerations. Oral Surg. 46:831, 1978

Winter GG, Brook AH: Enamel hypoplasia and anomalies of the enamel. Dent Clin North Am 19:3, 1975

Witkop CJ Jr: Hereditary defects of dentin. Dent Clin North Am 19:25, 1975

III. DISEASES OF THE TEETH AND SUPPORTING STRUCTURES

Abrams RA, Ruff JC; Oral signs and symptoms in diagnosis of bulimia. J Am Dent Assoc 113:761, 1986

Baume LJ: Biology of Pulp and Dentin. Basel & New York, S Karger AG, 1980

del Regato JA: Dental lesions observed after roentgen therapy in cancer of the buccal cavity, pharynx and larynx. Am J Roentgenol 42:404, 1939

Kerr D, Courtney R, Burkes EJ: Multiple idiopathic root resorption, Oral Surg 29:552, 1970

Lydiatt DD, Hollins RR, Peterson G: Multiple idiopathic root resorption: Diagnostic considerations. Oral Surg Oral Med Oral Pathol 67:208, 1989

Mandel ID: Dental caries. Am Sci 67:680, 1979

Mertz-Fairhurst EJ, Cella-Giustina VE, Brooks JE, Williams JE, Fairhurst CW: A comparative study of two pit and fissure sealants. J Am Dent Assoc 103:230, 1981

Primosch RE: Tetracycline discoloration, enamel defects, and dental caries in patients with cystic fibrosis. Oral Surg 50:301, 1980

Ripa LW: Fluoride rinsing: What every dentist should know. J Am Dent Assoc 102:477, 1981

Robinson HBG, Boling LR: Anachoretic effect in pulpitis. J Am Dent Assoc 28:268, 1941

Schrotenboer GH: Fluoride benefits after 36 years. J Am Dent Assoc 102:473, 1981

Seltzer S, Bender IB: The Dental Pulp, 3d ed. Philadelphia, JB Lippincott, 1984

Seltzer S: Endodontology, 2d ed. Philadelphia, Lea & Febiger, 1988.

Shaw J: Causes and control of dental caries. N Engl J Med 317:996, 1987

Westcott WB, Starcke EN, Shannon IL: Chemical protection against post-irradiation dental caries. Oral Surg 40:709, 1975

Wright JT, Grant DG: Epidermolysis bullosa associated with enamel hypoplasia and taurodontism. J Oral Pathol 12:73, 1983

Diseases of the Periodontium and Supporting Structures

Baer PN: Periodontosis (juvenile periodontitis): Differential diagnosis and treatment. In Richardson ER (ed): Periodontal Diseases in Children and Adolescents: State of the Art, Proceedings of a Symposium presented as a Part of the Dedication of the New Dental Facility, Meharry Medical College, Nashville, TN, May 21–23, 1979

Barak S, Engleberg I, Hiss J: Gingival hyperplasia caused by nifedipine: Histopathologic findings. J Periodontol 58:639, 1987

Clark RA, Page RC, Wilde G: Defective neutrophil chemotaxis in juvenile periodontitis. Infect Immun 18:694, 1977

Cuestas-Carnero R, Bornancini CA: Hereditary generalized gingival fibromatosis associated with hypertrichosis. J Oral Maxillofac Surg 46:415, 1988

Genco R, Slots J: Host responses in periodontal diseases. J Dent. Res 63:441, 1984

Hamner JE III, Scofield HH, Cornyn J: Benign fibro-osseous jaw lesions of periodontal membrane origin: Analysis of 249 cases. Cancer 22:861, 1968

Listgarten M: Pathogenesis of periodontitis. J Clin Periodontal 13:418, 1986

Meyer I: Osteoradionecrosis of the Jaws. Chicago, Year Book Medical Publishers, 1958

Murray CG, Daley TE, Zimmerman E: The relationship between dental disease and radiation necrosis of the mandible. Oral Surg 49:99, 1980

Rogers R, Sheridan P, Jordan R: Desquamative gingivitis. Clinical, histopathologic, and immunopathologic investigations. Oral Surg 42:316, 1976

Seymour GJ, Powell RN, Davies WIR: The immunopathogenesis of progressive chronic inflammatory periodontal disease J Oral Pathol 8:249, 1979

Slots J: The predominant cultivable organisms in juvenile periodontosis. Scand J Dent Res 84:1, 1976

IV. DISEASES OF THE ORAL SOFT TISSUES

Inflammatory, Infectious, and Reactive Conditions

Abrams AM, Melrose RJ, Howell FV: Necrotizing sialometaplasia: A disease simulating malignancy. Cancer 32:130, 1973

Adams HG: Herpes: A problem in older age groups. Geriatrics 38:91, 1983

Bhaskar SN, Beasley JD, Cutwright DE: Inflammatory hyperplasia of the oral mucosa: Report of 341 cases, J Am Dent Assoc 81:949, 1970

Buchner A, Hansen LS: The histomorphologic spectrum of peripheral ossifying fibroma. Oral Surg Oral Med Oral Pathol. 63:452, 1987

Cawson RA: Update on antiviral therapy: The advent of Acyclovir. Br Dent J 245:1986

Choukas NC, Toto PD, Condyloma acuminatum of the oral cavity. Oral Surg Oral Med Oral Pathol 54:480, 1982

Eversole LR: Oral sialocysts. Arch Otolarngol Head Neck Surg 113:5i, 1987

Eversole LR: Rovin S: Reactive lesions of the gingiva. J Oral Surg 27:716, 1969

Fujibasyashi T, Takahashi Y, Yoneda T, Tagami Y, Kusama M: Tuberculosis of the tongue: A case report with immunologic study. Oral Surg Oral Med Oral Pathol 47:427, 1979

Galasso GJ, Myers MW: The five human herpesviruses: Infection, prevention and treatment. Adv Intern Med 29:25, 1984

Giansanti JS, Waldron CA: Peripheral giant cell granuloma: Review of 720 cases. J Oral Surg 27:787, 1969

Jenson AB, Lancaster WD, Hartmann D-P, Shaffer EL Jr: Frequency and distribution of papillomavirus structural antigens in verrucae, multiple papillomas and condylomata of the oral cavity. Am J Pathol 107:212, 1982

Kostiala I: Acute fungal stomatitis in compromised host: causative agents, serological findings, topical treatment. Proc Finn Dent Soc 82 (suppl VIII): 1, 1986

Mani NJ: Secondary syphilis diagnosed from oral lesions. Oral Surg Oral Med Oral Pathol 58:47, 1984

Mintz GA, Rose SL: Diagnosis of oral herpes simplex infections: Practical aspects of viral culture. Oral Surg Oral Med Oral Pathol 58:486, 1984

Molinari JA, Sabes WR: Herpetic whitlow: A report of a case with multiple recurrences. Oral Surg Oral Med Oral Pathol 56:252, 1983

Morrish RB Jr, Chan E, Silverman S Jr, Meyer KK, Greenspan D: Osteonecrosis in patients irradiated for head and neck carcinoma. Cancer 47: 1981

Nazif MM, Ranalli DN: Stevens-Johnson syndrome: A report of 14 pediatric patients. Oral Surg Oral Med Oral Pathol 53:263, 1982

Schlossberg D (ed): Infections of the Head and Neck. New York, Springer-Verlag, 1987

Schroeder HE, Müller-Glauser W, Sallay K: Pathomorphologic features of the ulcerative stage of oral aphthous ulcerations. Oral Surg Oral Med Oral Pathol 58:293, 1984

Scully C, Prime S, Maitland N: Papillomaviruses: Their possible role in oral disease. Oral Surg Oral Med Oral Pathol 60:166, 1985

Sist TC, Green GW Jr: Traumatic neuromas of the oral cavity. Oral Surg 51:394, 1981

Wray D, Graykowski EA, Notkins AL: Role of mucosal injury in initiating recurrent aphthous stomatitis. Br Med J 283:1569, 1981

Mucosal White Patches and Red Patches

Bánóczy J, Roed-Petersen B, Pindborg JJ, Inovay J: Clinical and histologic studies on electrogalvanically induced oral white lesions. Oral Surg 45:319, 1979

Jorgenson RJ, Levin LS: White sponge nevus. Arch Dermatol 117:73, 1981

Kramer IRH, Lucas RB, Pindborg JJ, Sobin LH: Definition of leukoplakia and related lesions: An aid to studies on oral precancer. Oral Surg 46:518, 1978

Mackenzie IC, Dabelsteen E, Squier CA (eds): Oral Premalignancy. Proceedings of the First Dow's Symposium. Iowa City, University of Iowa Press, 1980

Mashberg A: Erythroplasia: The earliest sign of asympotomatic oral cancer. J Am Dent Assoc 96:616, 1978

Shafer WG, Waldron CA: Erythroplakia of the oral cavity. Cancer 36:1021, 1975

Waldron CA, Shafer WG: Leukoplakia revisited: A clinicopathologic study of 3,256 oral leukoplakias. Cancer 36:1386, 1975

Conditions Resulting From Altered Immune States

Antoon JW, Miller RL: Aphthous ulcers: A review of the literature on etiology, pathogenesis, diagnosis and treatment. J Am Dent Assoc 101:803, 1980

Daniels TE: Labial salivary gland biopsy in Sjögren's syndrome: Assessment as a diagnostic criterion in 362 suspected cases. Arthritis Rheumat 27:147, 1984

Ficarra G, Berson AM, Silverman S, et al.: Kaposi's sarcoma of the oral cavity: a study of 134 patients with a review of pathogenesis, epidemiology, clinical aspects, and treatment. Oral Surg Oral Med Oral Pathol 66:543, 1988

Foster ME, Nally FF: Benign mucous membrane pemphigoid (cicitrical mucosal pemphigoid): A reconsideration. Oral Surg 44:697, 1977

Goulet J-P: Immunofluorescence as a diagnostic aid in oral medicine, J Can Dent Assoc 53:217, 1987

Greenspan JS, Greenspan D, Pindborg JJ, Schiødt M: AIDS And the Dental Team. Chicago, Year Book Medical Publishers, 1986

Laskaris G, Sklavounou A, Stratigus J: Bullous pemphigoid, cicitrical pemphigoid and pemphigus vulgaris: A comparative survey of 278 cases. Oral Surg Oral Med Oral Pathol 54:656, 1982

Lozada-Nur F, Gorsky M, Silverman S: Oral erythema multiforme: Clinical observations and treatment of 95 patients. Oral Surg Oral Med Oral Pathol 67:36, 1989

Manton SL, Scully C: Mucous membrane pemphigoid: An elusive diagnosis? Oral Surg Oral Med Oral Pathol 66:37, 1988

Marmary Y, Glaiss, R, Pisanty S: Scleroderma: Oral manifestations. Oral Surg Oral Med Oral Pathol 52:32, 1981

McCarthy PL, Shklar G: Diseases of the Oral Mucosa, 2d ed. Philadelphia, Lea & Febiger, 1980

Phelan JA, Saltzman BR, Friedland GH, Klein RS: Oral findings in patients with AIDS. Oral Surg Oral Med Oral Pathol 64:50, 1987

Schiødt M, Greenspan D, Daniels TE, Greenspan JS: Clinical and histologic spectrum of oral hairy leukoplakia. Oral Surg Oral Med Oral Pathol 64:716, 1987

Schiødt M, Pindborg JJ: Epidemiology and clinical oral manifestations of human immune deficiency virus infection: A review. Int J Oral Maxillofac Surg 16:1, 1987

Scully C: Sjögren's syndrome: Clinical and laboratory features, immunopathogenesis, and management. Oral Surg Oral Med Oral Pathol 62:510, 1986

Zegarelli DJ, Zegarelli EV: Intraoral pemphigus vulgaris. Oral Surg 44:384, 1977

V. NON-NEOPLASTIC CONDITIONS OF THE JAW BONES

Airienne P: X-linked hypohidrotic ectodermal dysplasia in Finland. Proc Finn Dent Soc 77 (suppl 1):7, 1981

Barker BF, Jensen JL, Howell FV: Focal osteoporotic bone marrow defects of the jaws. Oral Surg 38:404, 1974

Ellis G, Connole P: Diffuse mandibular enlargement caused by osteitis deformans. Ear Nose Throat J 64:466, 1985

Ficarra G, Kaban LB, Hansen LS: Central giant cell lesions of the mandible and maxilla: A clinicopathologic and cytometric study. Oral Surg Oral Med Oral Pathol 64:44, 1987

Hamner JE, Ketcham AS: Cherubism: An analysis of treatment. Cancer 23:1113, 1969

Hartman KS: Histiocytosis X: Review of 114 cases with oral involvement. Oral Surg 49:38, 1980

Jacobsson, S: Diffuse sclerosing osteomyelitis of the mandible. Int J Oral Surg 13:363, 1984

Kaugars GE, Cale AE: Traumatic bone cyst. Oral Surg Oral Med Oral Pathol 63:318, 1987

Lipani CS, Natiella JR, Greene GW: Hematopoietic defect of jaws: Report of 16 cases. J Oral Pathol 11:411, 1982

Osband, ME, Lipton JM, et al: Histiocytosis X: Demonstration of abnormal immunity, T-cell histamine H2-receptor deficiency, and successful treatment with thymic extract. N Engl J Med 304:146, 1981

Schneider LC, Mesa ML, Fraenkel D: Osteoporotic bone marrow defect: Radiographic features and pathogenic factors. Oral Surg Oral Med Oral Pathol 65:127, 1988

Schweiger JW: Oral complications following radiation therapy: A five-year retrospective study. J Prosth Dent 58:78, 1987

Stewart JCB, Regezi JA, Lloyd RV, McClatchey KD: Immunohistochemical study of idiopathic histiocytosis of the mandible and maxilla. Oral Surg Oral Med Oral Pathol 61:48, 1986

Waldron CA: Fibro-osseous lesions of the jaws. J Oral Maxillofac Surg 43:249, 1985

Waldron CA, Giansanti JS: Benign fibro-osseous lesions of the jaws. Part I: Fibrous dysplasia of the jaws. Oral Surg 35:190, 1973

Waldron CA, Giansanti JS: Benign fibro-osseous lesions of the jaws: A clinical-radiologic-histologic review of sixty-five cases. Part II: Benign fibro-osseous lesions of periodontal ligament origin. Oral Surg 35:340, 1973

Zachariades N, Papanicolaou S, Xypolyta A, et al: Cherubism. Int J Oral Surg 14:138, 1985

VI. GENETIC, METABOLIC AND ENDOCRINE DISTURBANCES

Antoniades K, Eleftheriades I, Karakasis D: The Gardner syndrome. Int J Oral Maxillofac Surg 16:480, 1987

Austin GB, Quart AM, Novak B: Hereditary hemorrhagic telangiectasia with oral manifestations. Oral Surg 51:245, 1981

Buchner A, Hansen LS: Pigmented nevi of the oral mucosa: A clinicopathologic study of 36 new cases and review of 155 cases from the literature. Part II: Analysis of 191 cases. Oral Surg Oral Med Oral Pathol 63:676, 1987

Dummett CO: Normal pigmentation of oral soft tissues. Quintessence Int 10:1032, 1979

Flint SR, Keith O, Scully C: Hereditary hemorrhagic telangiectasia: Family study and review. Oral Surg Oral Med Oral Pathol 66:440, 1988

Jarvis JL, Keats TE: Cleidocranial dysostosis: A review of 40 new cases. Am J Roentgenol 121:5, 1974

Luk GD, Gaylin SB: Ornithine decarboxylase as a biologic marker in familial polyposis. N Engl J Med 311:80, 1984

Miller CS, Craig, RM Jr: White corrugated mucosa. J Am Dent Assoc 117:345, 1988

VII. NEOPLASMS

General References

Batsakis JG: Tumors of the Head and Neck, 2nd ed. Baltimore, Williams & Wilkins, 1979

Field JK, Spandidos DA: Expression of oncogenes in human tumors with special reference to the head and neck, J Oral Pathol 16:97, 1987

Robinson HBG (ed): Tumors of the Oral Regions. Philadelphia, WB Saunders, 1957

Rosai J: Ackerman's Surgical Pathology, 7th ed. St. Louis, CV Mosby, 1989

Stout AP, Lattes R: Atlas of Tumor Pathology, 2nd series, Fascicle I: Tumors of the Soft Tissues. Washington, DC, Armed Forces Institute of Pathology, 1966

Salivary Gland Neoplasms

Evans RW, Cruickshank AH: Major Problems in Pathology, Vol 1. Epithelial Tumors of the Salivary Glands. Philadelphia, WB Saunders, 1970

Eveson JW, Cawson RA: Salivary gland tumors: A review of 2,410 cases with particular reference to histologic types, site, age, and sex distribution. J Pathol 146:51, 1985

Mason DK, Chisholm DM: Salivary Glands in Health and Disease. London, Philadelphia, WB Saunders, 1975

McKenna RJ: Tumors of major and minor salivary glands. CA 34:24, 1984

O'Brien, CJ, Soong, S-J, Herrera GA, Urist MM, Maddox WA: Malignant salivary tumors: An analysis of prognostic factors and survival. Head Neck Surg. 9:82, 1986

Thackery AC, Lucas RB: Atlas of Tumor Pathology, 2nd series, Fascicle 10: Tumors of the Major Salivary Glands. Washington, DC, Armed Forces Institute of Pathology, 1974

Benign Soft Tissue Neoplasms

Green TL, Eversole LR, Leider AS: Oral and labial verruca vulgaris: Clinical, histologic, and immunohistochemical evaluation. Oral Surg Oral Med Oral Pathol 62:410, 1986

Ostberg Y: Clinical picture of benign lymphoepithelial lesion. Clin Otolaryngol 8:381, 1983

Wright JM, Dunsworth AR: Follicular lymphoid hyperplasia of the hard palate: A benign lymphoproliferative process. Oral Surg Oral Med Oral Pathol 55:162, 1983

Zhao-ju Z Yun-Tang W, Guang-xui S, Xian-zhong Z, Zhong-qi H: Clinical application of angiography of oral and maxillofacial hemangiomas. Oral Surg Oral Med Oral Pathol 55:437, 1983

Oral Squamous Cell Carcinoma

DeCroix, Y, Chesseim NA: Experience in the Curie Institute in treatment of cancer of the mobile tongue. Part I: Treatment policies and results. Cancer 47:496, 1981

Farr HW, Goldfarb PM, Farr CN: Epidermoid carcinoma of the mouth and pharynx at Memorial Sloan-Kettering Cancer Center, 1965–1969. Am J Surg 140:563, 1980

Schantz SP, Byers RM, Goepfert H, Shallenberger RC, Beddingfield N: The implication of tobacco use in the young adult with head and neck cancer. Cancer 62:1374, 1988

Shafer WG: Oral carcinoma in situ. Oral Surg 39:227, 1975

Silverman S Jr, Griffith M: Smoking characteristics of patients with oral carcinoma and risk for second oral primary carcinoma. J Am Dent Assoc 85:637, 1972

Son YH, Kapp OS: Oral cavity and oropharyngeal cancer in a younger population: Review of literature and experience at Yale. Cancer 55:441, 1985

Thoma GW: Cause of death in patients with oral cancer. Oral Surg 30:817, 1970

Malignant Lymphoma

Howell RE, Handlers JP, Abrams AM, Melrose RJ: Extranodal oral lymphoma. Part II: Relationships between clinical features and the Lukes-Collins classification of 34 cases. Oral Surg Oral Med Oral Pathol 64:597, 1987

Hupp JR, Collins FJV, Ross A, Myall RWT: Review of Burkitt's lymphoma: Importance of radiographic diagnosis. J Oral Maxillofac Surg 10:240, 1982

Tomich CE, Shafer WG: Lymphoproliferative disease of the hard palate: A clinicopathologic entity. Oral Surg 39:754, 1975

Multiple Myeloma

Gross PD, Roth NA, Koudelka BM: Multiple myeloma presenting as a hemorrhagic diathesis. J Oral Maxillofac Surg 4:125, 1983

Odontogenic Neoplasms

Courtney RM, Kerr DA: Odontogenic adenomatoid tumors: Comprehensive study of 20 new cases. Oral Surg 39:424, 1975

Eversole LR, Leider AS, Strub D: Radiographic characteristics of cystogenic ameloblastoma. Oral Surg Oral Med Oral Pathol 57:572, 1984

Kaugers GE, Miller ME, Abbey LM: Odontomas. Oral Surg Oral Med Oral Pathol 67:172, 1989

Lucas RB: Pathology of Tumours of the Oral Tissues, 2nd ed. Baltimore, Williams & Wilkins, 1972

Melrose RJ, Abrams AM, Mills BG: Florid osseous dysplasia: A clinical-pathologic study of thirty-four cases. Oral Surg 41:62, 1976

Pindborg JJ: Calcifying epithelial odontogenic tumor: Review of literature and report of an extraosseous case. Acta Odontol Scand 4:419, 1966

Pindborg JJ, Kramer IRH: Histologic Typing of Odontogenic Tumors, Jaws Cysts, and Related Lesions. Geneva, World Health Organization, 1971

Regezi JA, Kerr DA, Courtney RM: Odontogenic tumors: Analysis of 706 cases. J Oral Surg 36:771, 1978

Slootweg PJ, Wittkampf ARM: Myxoma of the jaws: An analysis of 15 cases. J Oral Maxillofac Surg 14:46, 1986

Trodahl JN: Ameloblastic fibroma: A survey of cases from the Armed Forces Institute of Pathology. Oral Surg 33:547, 1972

White DK, Chen S-Y, Mohnac AM, Miller AS: Odontogenic myxoma: Clinical and ultrastructural study. Oral Surg 39:901, 1975

Waldron CA, El-Mofty SK: A histopathologic study of 116 ameloblastomas with special reference to the desmoplastic variant. Oral Surg Oral Med Oral Pathol 63:441, 1987

Woolgar JA, Rippen JW, Browne RM: A comparative histologic study of odontogenic keratocysts in basal cell nevus syndrome. J Oral Pathol 16:75, 1987

Melanoma

Eckhardt A: Primary malignant melanoma of the oral mucosa. J Oral Maxillofac Surg 45:1068, 1987

Jackson D, Simpson HC: Primary melanoma of the oral cavity. Oral Surg 39:553, 1975

Rapini RP, Golitz LE, Greer RO Jr, Krekorian EA, Poulson T: Primary melanoma of the oral cavity: A review of 177 cases. Cancer 55:1543, 1985

Regezi JA, Hayward JR, Pickens TN: Superficial melanoma of oral mucous membranes. Oral Surg 45:730, 1978

Takagi M, Ishikawa G, Mori W: Primary malignant melanoma of the oral cavity in Japan with special reference to mucosal melanomatosis. Cancer 34:358, 1974

Sarcoma

Ajagbe HA, Daramola JO, Junaid TA: Chondrosarcoma of the jaws: Review of fourteen cases. J Oral Maxillofac Surg 43:763, 1985

Russ JE, Jesse RN: Management of osteosarcoma of the maxilla and mandible. Am J Surg 140:572, 1980

Metastasis to Oral Structures

Castigliano SG, Romiger CJ: Metastatic malignancy of the jaws. Am J Surg 87:496, 1954

Cherrick HM, Demkee D: Metastatic carcinoma of the jaws. J Am Dent Assoc 17:180, 1973

Kaugars GE, Svirsky JA: Lung malignancies metastatic to the oral cavity. Oral Surg 51:197, 1981

Keller EE, Gunderson LL: Bone disease metastatic to the jaws. J Am Dent Assoc 115:697, 1987

Vider M, Maruyama Y, Narvaez R: Significance of the vertebral venous (Batson's) plexus in metastatic spread in colorectal carcinoma. Cancer 40:67, 1977

Index

ISBN 0-397-51043-8

9 780397 510436

90000